W0038375

Dr Dhurandhar's Fat-loss Diet

Dear Dr. Mali,

I hope that you get to enjoy this book.

With Best Wishes

– N.V. Dhurandhar
El Paso, TX
Dec 7, 2018

Dr Nikhil V. Dhurandhar

HarperCollins *Publishers* India

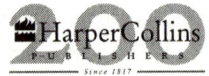

First published in India by
HarperCollins *Publishers* in 2017
A-75, Sector 57, Noida, Uttar Pradesh 201301, India
www.harpercollins.co.in

2 4 6 8 10 9 7 5 3 1

Copyright © Syndicated Wellness LLC

P-ISBN: 978-93-5277-030-4
E-ISBN: 978-93-5277-031-1

The views and opinions expressed in this book are the author's own and the facts are
as reported by him, and the publishers are not in any way liable for the same.

Dr Nikhil V. Dhurandhar asserts the moral right
to be identified as the author of this work.

All rights reserved. No part of this publication may be reproduced,
stored in a retrieval system, or transmitted, in any form or by any means,
electronic, mechanical, photocopying, recording or otherwise,
without the prior permission of the publishers.

Typeset in 11/14 Bembo Std at
Manipal Digital Systems, Manipal

Printed and bound at
Thomson Press (India) Ltd.

Dr Dhurandhar's Fat-loss Diet

Dr Nikhil V. Dhurandhar, is a physician and nutritional biochemist who has been involved in obesity treatment for thirty-five years. He started his weight management practice in Mumbai, learning first-hand from his father – Dr Vinod Dhurandhar, the founding father of obesity medicine in India. Since then, he has helped about 15,000 patients lose weight.

As a scientist, he has written 135 scientific articles, and given over 200 scientific presentations. He has received fourteen patents for inventions, which led to his induction to the National Academy of Inventors (USA). For his weight management practice and research, he has received many prestigious awards, including from Nutrition Society of India, and the American Society of Nutrition.

He is a Professor and Chairman of the department of Nutritional Sciences at Texas Tech University. He is a past president of The Obesity Society (USA), and a founding member of the All India Association for Advancing Research in Obesity.

His life and work have been featured by numerous media outlets, including *Times of India*, *Indian Express*, *New York Times*, National Geographic, BBC-UK, CNN. He was listed in the '30 Best and Brightest Minds in the U.S.' by *Esquire* magazine. Find more information about him at: www.dhurandhar.com.

Contents

Contents

Foreword

When I started work on *Dangal* I knew I would have to go through a major body transformation. This would require a great trainer, a lot of hard work and focus from me, but more importantly, I would need a first-rate nutritionist. This last requirement I was not worried about because I had worked with Dr Vinod Dhurandhar in the past, always achieving great results.

I began putting on the weight and then it occurred to me that even as I was putting on weight it might be a good idea to warn Dr Vinod Dhurandhar that this is what I was up to, and that in the near future I was going to come to him to help me get back into shape. With that in mind I called up his clinic. I tried for several days but I just could not get through. I had Dr Vinod Dhurandhar's cell number but I was hesitant to call on that. However, after trying his clinic in vain for almost a month I thought I should try his personal number.

The phone was answered by his wife Mrs Anuradha Dhurandhar. She told me that Dr Vinod was rather unwell, and that as a result of his bad health there was no way that he could meet me and nor could he help me professionally. I was of course very sad to hear that Dr Vinod was so unwell. He had helped so many thousands like me. I expressed my regrets to Mrs Dhurandhar and put the phone down.

Over the next few days I was getting more and more anxious about who I should consult on my diet plan and nutrition. What I was attempting in this film was a very big challenge, and Dr Vinod Dhurandhar was the only person whom I trusted to help me achieve this near impossible task of first putting on 25-30 kgs, and then losing it in a short span of time.

I called Mrs Dhurandhar again, this time to ask if she could recommend to me any of Dr Vinod's assistants who could perhaps help me. No name came to her immediately, but she said she would give it a thought and get back.

I waited, wondering what to do next. I had already reached 85 kgs by now and was well on my way to achieve my 'fat look', but I still did not have a person who would help me get back in shape. I felt a little like Abhimanyu who broke into the Chakravyuha but did not have the knowledge to break out of it.

Two days later I got a call from Dr Dhurandhar's cell, only it wasn't Mrs Dhurandhar on the line. Instead, a gentle, well-spoken male voice asked to speak with me. This was Dr Nikhil

Dhurandhar, son of Dr Vinod Dhurandhar. Turns out that he was in Mumbai to see his ailing father (Dr Nikhil lives in the US), and his mother had spoken to him about my call.

'Mr Khan, I no longer make diets for people, instead I am doing research in obesity, but at one time I used to. In fact, I worked along with my father for a good ten years a long time ago. I am aware of your professional relationship with my father, he often mentioned you as his favourite patient. Therefore, if you like, as a one off, I can try and help you.'

You can imagine how relieved I was to hear this! We met two days later in my house.

Dr Nikhil is a conservative man. And that's coming from me!

He heard out my absurd requirement patiently and then gave me his reaction. 'Mr Khan, this is rather a strange requirement, not to mention difficult. I must confess I have never done something like this before. Also, I must warn you that what you are attempting is very difficult.' For the entire remainder of the meeting he proceeded to warn me in different ways how near impossible the task I had set for myself. He pointed out that age was not on my side. He warned me that losing weight was not simple math, it was biology, and every person reacts differently and to different extents. On and on he went about how it was a daunting task. He was willing to take on the challenge but was assuring me nothing save that it was going to be very difficult. I liked him immediately. I trust people who are conservative and who hesitate to promise results. The other quality I liked about him was that he is a man of detail. I felt I was in safe hands. I needed someone who is realistic and whose knowledge is thorough. I knew I was going to give it all but I needed someone guiding me in nutrition who I could trust blindly. I did not want to put in effort barking up the wrong tree.

I had found my man.

We set the date for starting out. I told him it would be after I had finished shooting for the fat part, so it was still months away.

Then the time finally arrived. I had almost finished shooting for the fat part and was ready to start the fat loss process in a few weeks. At that time I stood at 97 kgs and 38 per cent body fat. I told Dr Nikhil the time had come. Of course, he wanted a lot of tests done before he gave me a diet; he needed to know my health parameters. The most fundamental principle that both Dr Dhurandhar senior and junior follow is that they are not just giving you a diet for fat loss, their diet also addresses any health issues you may have like high cholesterol, high BP, diabetes, etc. So, the fat loss programme is centred around good health.

We decided to follow a system of communication since we were in different countries. Every week on Sunday morning I would do detailed measurements of myself and send them to him. Every Sunday I would also give him a details of how accurate I had been with the diet. So, he would have a weekly progress report from me. Based on that, whenever necessary, he would change the diet. Also, he would change the diet when I felt I am getting too used to a particular pattern of eating.

I remember when I started out on the fat loss I had three weeks off from work. I asked him if he could find me a place where I could go to for this period, like a health resort. Some place where I would have no other distractions. He did his research and came up with the ideal place, Canyon Ranch in Arizona. Because of the various physical activities available there, I was able to reach a daily calorie deficit of 2,500 calories! I was spending 8 hrs a day doing some physical activity or the other. Three hrs hike up the mountain, 1 hr weight training, 1 hr swimming/water aerobics, 90 mins tennis, 2 hrs cycling, 90 mins walking. This was intense and we decided that this I would do for just three weeks as a strong start to the process.

We were off to a good start. However, somewhere around the two-and-a-half month mark, back in Mumbai, I felt that I had begun slipping. I had begun to see results and I was getting tempted with eating things which were out of my diet plan. I was succumbing to temptation, my resolve was getting weak. After a couple of weeks of stumbling I spoke to Dr Nikhil about it. He asked me what would help me to stick to the diet. I said, a more regular contact with him. We decided a method where I would text him every day after every meal. For example, I would text him at 7 a.m. that I just ate my breakfast, what it was exactly that I ate, and I would also tell him that my next meal was at 9 a.m. and was 100gm of papaya and one scoop of protein shake in water. Then at 9.15 a.m. I would text him that I ate my fruit and protein shake and my next meal was at 11 a.m. and was one toast and 25gm of tuna and 1/4 cup of slim yogurt. All this while he was asleep in the US. He would wake up and check my texts and send me an encouraging message. This constant reporting after every meal helped me get back on to track.

In five months, and exactly one day before my shoot for the younger Mahaveer Phogat, I had reached 80 kg and 9.67 per cent body fat. I was heavier than my usual 70 kgs but that was because I was very muscular and muscle weighs much more than fat. Importantly I was looking exactly as I wanted to.

Not only is Dr Nikhil a very solid nutritionist, but I also found him to be extremely supportive and helpful. Thanks Doc for helping me achieve what you repeatedly warned me was very difficult.

I wish Dr Nikhil all the very best for this book. I can't think of a better person to help readers understand about good nutrition. I hope that readers all across the world can benefit from his knowledge in the field of nutrition.

Wish all of you a good read, and good health.

Cheers
Aamir

1

Why Am I Fat?

'I know why I am fat,' said Ms Bina, my final patient on a Friday night in March. 'We got married in November and for three straight months after the honeymoon I enjoyed going for a scooter ride with my husband every night. It was the winter and all that cold air got trapped in my body and I ballooned. Please, help me get rid of that air from my body.' This is a true story. Clearly Ms Bina was misinformed. Most of you probably know that you don't gain fat from cold air filling you up, yet you may be wondering: why *does* someone gain fat and, more importantly, why is it so hard to lose that fat and then keep it off? I bet you have heard your share of theories about what causes obesity and what helps in its treatment. One oft-repeated refrain being, 'All the tasty food that you are eating is causing your obesity', or 'You are fat because you are greedy and lazy.'

Let me say this loud and clear – food does not 'cause' obesity, nor does greediness or laziness. Surprised? There is more. From now on, forget the words 'weight loss'. It is 'fat loss' that you should be thinking about. Obesity needs a specific and strategic treatment plan because just trying to eat healthier and exercising more will not address the obesity concerns of most people. Furthermore, it is not true that to keep from regaining fat you should live like a sanyasi, giving up all the good things in life like tasty food and drinks and survive on only salads. Sounds strange to you? Well, it is time for you to get acquainted with modern scientific concepts.

For decades, my team and I have conducted cutting-edge research in obesity as well as worked and interacted with highly respected researchers in the field of obesity. Many of the theories that your nutritionists or doctors may have told you have been discovered by the same researchers I have had the pleasure of calling my colleagues, or discovered in my lab. For example, you may have heard the recent news that eggs are very good for weight loss because they quickly fill you up. I am proud to say that my team was the first in the world to discover this.

This book has not been written by a self-proclaimed 'nutritionist' with no real qualifications, full of feel-good or provocative nutrition theories written in a fact-free zone. To help you understand the truth about weight loss, I will translate the experience and knowledge I have gained from my Masters in nutrition, my medical degree, my PhD in biochemistry and my medical treatment for obesity of over 15,000 patients, and the twenty-five years of evidence-based research and discoveries my colleagues and I have made in the field of obesity. This is who I am, and here is my story.

Big Fat Lies

In 1982, I graduated from medical school. I had decided, quite early on, that I was going to follow in my father's footsteps. Dr Vinod Dhurandhar was India's first obesity physician – a trailblazer. He started his practice in 1962. By the 1980s, he was swamped with patients seeking obesity treatment. This was in part because of his growing reputation, but also because rates of obesity were skyrocketing.

The stories he told at the dinner table motivated me as a child. He related to us the plight of people with obesity. Along with my father's booming practice, many other self-described weight loss 'experts' put up their hoardings in Mumbai. Desperate people with a real medical condition were seeking help wherever they could, and being swindled and cheated by quacks who sold nonsense cures.

As I entered practice in 1982, I imagined that the days of 'quackery' were over. I thought that the phony treatments may have worked back in the day but surely patients were more informed now. How little I knew!

In my first month of practice, a woman walked into the clinic. Her name was Sneha. As I do with all my patients, I asked her about her medical history, current health status and other factors such as family medical history and her struggles with weight management. When I asked about her past attempts to diet, she said, 'Doctor, I have tried every diet imaginable. I have been to every dietitian in Mumbai.'

'Are you on any diet now?'

She thought it through and said, 'No, not at the moment. I'm seeing a doctor, but she is not giving me a diet.'

'What is she giving you?'

'It's a fat-breaking treatment.'

I nodded and jotted down 'fat-breaking treatment'. It was just my first month as a practitioner and I had already lost track of all the 'treatments' patients would tell me about. Almost none of them were real treatments that worked. This fat-breaking treatment was going to be an addition to the list.

One of the elements of a physical exam is blood pressure measurement. Blood pressure tells us the condition of a patient's heart. It's measured by wrapping a cloth cuff around the upper arm and inflating it with a pump. As I measured her blood pressure, I noticed she had blue-black marks on her arm. Bruises. She had been beaten.

My mind instantly went to a thousand dark places. She was married. Was it her husband? Was she a victim of spousal abuse? How could I help her? Should I report it to police? I asked her, 'What happened, ma'am? How did you get these bruises?'

'Oh!' she said, gently rubbing the bruise, 'It only hurts a little.'

I pressed on, 'How did you get them?'

'From my dietician.'

'Your *dietician*?'

'Um, yes.'

'What did your dietitian do to you?'

'She beat me with a cricket bat!'

'What?' I yelled. 'why would she do that?'

She looked at me confused. 'Don't you know, doctor?'

I shook my head.

She moved her sari slightly and revealed large bruises on her abdomen.

'Well, she beats me – it's the fat breaking treatment. She says it is necessary to first break down the accumulated fat with a bat, only then will I be able to lose it.'

I was wrong about the quacks. A decade after my father encountered them, they were still thriving and cheating people. The 'cricket bat treatment' doesn't work. It is physically impossible to 'break down' fat from outside of the body. Not only was this treatment fraudulent, but my patient was lucky to have survived it. At worst, this kind of beating can lead to internal bleeding and death.

This single story is indeed sorrowful and there will always be quacks taking advantage of gullible people. Why are such practices accepted by patients as 'treatments'? The answer is desperation. Patients are desperate. They are so desperate, they are willing to be beaten black and blue with cricket bats, as long as it will help them lose weight. Many of you reading this book may have been at this point. Many of you may have undergone extreme diets, extreme treatments and extreme teasing. For some of you, perhaps your entire life. I am writing this book for you, and I have incredible news to share.

We all want to reach a point where our weight is not a concern. But before we reach there, we've got to understand how we got *here*. The first question I want to answer for you is a question you may have pondered upon after having failed a diet, sweating in the gym or waking up at night craving food: Why am I fat?

'Why am I fat?'

Here's the answer: it's our ancestors' fault. The human species evolved in times of desperate famine. Our ancestors, since humans evolved, ate only on the days they could successfully hunt a deer or find some fruits. And the days when they found sustenance were rare. How did they survive the days in between? The secret: fat. Their bodies stored fat the way a car stores petrol in the tank.

There must have been some early humans who could not store fat very well. Most of them must have simply perished during lean times, leaving no offspring. So, we are here because our ancestors had the ability to survive *between* days of food as their bodies burned up stored fat for the energy needed to walk, breathe and think. Therefore, the need to store fat is deeply rooted in the ability of humans to survive. Food consumption is needed to build these fat reserves for a rainy day. It is little surprise then that food is such an important part of our lives.

Think about the last time you went to a restaurant. What was the purpose of going out to eat? Few us would say that treating yourself to a lavish meal is necessary for *survival*. Most of us would agree that going out is about unwinding and socializing, not sustenance. Consider how strange a concept this is! Food is eaten for sustenance. But why have we built a culture around it? Why does it give us pleasure to eat, even when not hungry?

The fact is, this behaviour of seeking food, enjoying it in ways that are disconnected from sustenance, has helped human beings survive. We survived famines because our traditions emphasize the acquisition of food and making it tasty and enjoyable. Our societies and cultures have evolved around these concepts. We all love to eat for pleasure because our bodies are designed to eat for pleasure. We cannot help it. Sex is similar. Nature wants us to procreate. Sex allows us to procreate. Making sex pleasurable ensures that human beings will engage in sex and procreate.

But, here's the problem about food nowadays – except in rare circumstances, we do not live in famine today. Most of us reading this book live in a world of plenty. Delicious food, high in fat (which is incidentally why food tastes good), is available at the snap of a finger. We have access to quantities and varieties of food our ancestors could not even dream of. Yet, our drive to seek food has remained the same. This has complicated nature's job of fat accumulation.

Nature ensures that fat storage is not too much nor too little as both cases result in several ill effects. If a woman has too little fat, nature considers it as a sign that she may not be able to support a pregnancy. As a result, pregnancy becomes very difficult. On the other extreme, excess fat can also result in problems with conception, complications during pregnancy and birthing and even birth defects. And how, you may wonder, does our body track fat and control its accumulation? The whole process is quite complex, but it is easy to understand with some simple examples. Body fat makes a chemical named leptin, which travels to the brain via the bloodstream. Too little leptin signals to the brain that there is too little fat in the body whereas too much leptin means too much fat. The lesser your brain receives leptin, the more your brain makes you eat. Whereas, if you have too much fat, the brain notices too much leptin, tries to make you eat less, so you could lose some fat.

So, what translates the brain's desire to make you eat less or more? One answer is: ghrelin. Ghrelin is the name of a tiny chemical messenger (a hormone) that is made by the gut and generates the feeling of hunger. The hormone tells the brain it is 'time to eat'. Without ghrelin, we would never feel hungry or seek out food, and possibly starve. For some of us, however, the problem is not *starting* to eat, but rather, *stopping*. And, brain knows how to address that issue too. Another hormone named PYY (peptide tyrosine tyrosine), tells your brain when the stomach is full and stops you from eating further. I suppose you are getting the picture. Our free will can still overrule the brain signals and we may eat even when the brain signal says we are full, or refuse to eat, even when the signal is that we are hungry. In summary, leptin conveys to the brain whether the body has too much fat stored, or if it needs more fat. In response, the brain manipulates the hunger and fullness hormones accordingly to make you eat more or reduce your eating. These manipulations of the hormones go on in the body without your active knowledge and drive you to eat more, or less. Next time you want to blame someone for feeling hungry and eating more than you do, think of these messengers.

You are probably thinking, 'If the brain can control hunger and fullness and body fat accumulation, why do some people have normal fat stores while others have too much? Should the brain not keep all of us in a normal range of body fat?' The answer to this question holds the secret to understanding obesity. In many people, the body indeed keeps fat storage under check. Surely, you know people who remain slim lifelong. In some people, however, this control does not work as perfectly. For example, remember leptin, the hormone that reports body fat amount to brain? Some people are born without the ability to make any leptin. As a result, their brain does not 'see' leptin. Naturally, even though they have fat, the brain thinks that they have no fat stores and need to accumulate. In these individuals, the brain encourages one to keep eating. They get fat right from childhood and stay that way (but remember that not all obesity in children is due to this cause).

Another reason is when the hunger or fullness hormones are malfunctioning. You can imagine the result when someone is born with the tendency to produce too much PPY or ghrelin. There is more. Beyond controlling food intake, our bodies can also burn off excess food that is eaten. Some people are born with the blessing that when they eat excess food, their body simply burns off that excess. And then, there are also those people whose bodies are not that good at burning excess food, which gets stored in the body in the form of fat. Shocking as it is, in one sense we are puppets in the hands of the puppet master: our biology.

The 'Skinny' on Fat

Many carefully conducted scientific studies have shown that our ability to store body fat varies widely. The participants of these scientific studies were intentionally overfed huge amounts of food (of course, after obtaining their consent). Even in response to the same amount of overfeeding, some people gain very little fat, if any, while others gain a lot of fat. It is because of their differing biology. Now, we begin to see how superficial it is to blame a person's obesity on the food they eat. Obesity is due to anomalies in biology. Food does not cause these differences in a person's biology. Further chapters of this book will also reveal other causes of obesity, including certain infections that can lead to excess fat accumulation.

In asking the question, 'Why am I fat?' an implied question is, 'What could I do to lose fat'? This book is written to answer this very question. But before getting there, it is equally important for us to know what you should *not* do to lose fat. And, where should we begin? There is a long list of things that you may have heard from your friends, neighbours, or at times even from some doctors, dietitians or nutritionists that may be completely useless and at times downright harmful. Some build unsupported theories around a grain of truth and some are out-and-out shameless scams.

I remember one such example. I had gone to the beautiful seaside resort of Cancun, Mexico, for a conference on obesity. Incidentally, I was watching TV in my hotel room. A programme on weight loss on one channel caught my attention. It was about a soap for weight loss. The person conducting the programme was confidently and convincingly selling a bath soap that you use while showering. The soap gets all your fat out and washes it away. I wanted to yell at those quacks in the TV. How? How does the soap get that fat out of the body? Does it simply ooze out of skin pores like sweat? This baseless theory was being presented by good-looking models in a well-made infomercial. How could one *not* fall for something so polished? Well, what it would take to not be fooled by such a lie, is the true knowledge of how one loses fat. So, let's see just how that happens.

The purpose of storing fat in the body is much like why a car stores petrol in a petrol tank: to use it for producing energy. When does this petrol in the tank reduce? It is reduced when the car uses that petrol for running the engine. You cannot reduce the petrol levels by rubbing the petrol tank from outside or wrapping the tank in warm blankets, or for that matter, using a soap. Much the same way, the stored fat in your body decreases only when your body uses it for running its engine, i.e., for producing energy. So, no vibrating belts, no body massages, kneading various body parts, or beating with a cricket bat, is going to do a thing. I have often heard the expression 'melting the fat away'. This is also a misnomer. Your body is not a freezer. At body temperature, fat exists in a liquid state and does not need any 'melting'.

Next time you hear that taking a steam bath or sauna bath will melt your fat away, rest assured that the person may be intentionally misleading you, or maybe he is well-meaning but ill informed. A steam or a sauna bath may make you feel refreshed and that is all. If you weigh yourself before and after a sauna bath, you may notice that you have lost some weight. Before you are sold on this too easy a way of losing fat, note the real gimmick. These baths make you perspire. Thus, you lose water from the body. All that weight loss you noticed is simply due to loss of water. Drink a few glasses of water and your weight is back. All of it.

This leads us to the next important point. Weight loss versus fat loss. If your excess body weight is due to excess fat, would you not aim to reduce that excess fat? Why then would the quacks peddle remedies for that make you pass more urine, or laxatives to relieve constipation, under the guise of reducing obesity? It is because they are counting on the fact that by passing more urine, or getting rid of accumulated waste from intestines, you would weigh less. Yet, you will readily see that such loss of weight is not loss of fat. This is similar to losing weight by steam or sauna bath. Weight loss, yes. Fat loss, no!

I remember that many years ago, a company appeared in Mumbai and other places, promising instant reduction in weight and body measurements. Its shiny offices, lab coat-wearing staff and full-page ads in prominent newspapers were generating buzz. Surely, they must knew some secret, right? Their treatment: to wrap your body in a tight bandage and put you in a suit made of polyethylene-like material. The result: measurable loss of weight and inches right after each session lasting several minutes. What a miracle. Painless weight loss was finally here. But, here comes the sad part. The whole process was a gimmick. By tightly compressing the body in bandages, you temporarily reduce body measurement, much the same as the mark left on your wrist after wearing a wristwatch too tight. The body suit made one perspire profusely. Due to that loss of water, people lost weight right after the session. The only actual 'slimming' was of their customers' wallets.

There is one more reason to be mindful of the difference between weight loss and fat loss. On a diet, your weight loss is due to loss of fat and muscle mass. Fat loss is desirable; muscle loss is not. The type of diet and exercise plan you follow can impact how much of the weight lost is due to fat and muscles. Usually, diets that are extremely low in calories or proteins will result in a large proportion of muscle loss. By carefully planning a diet, the muscle loss could be minimized and fat loss increased. A familiar example is of the Bollywood superstar, Aamir Khan, who lost weight under my guidance for his movie, *Dangal*.

In the movie, Khan plays the role of an elderly, overweight, former champion wrestler, as well as his incredibly fit younger self. This younger look required him to lose body fat to an incredible 10 per cent and to gain big muscles fit for a wrestler. In several months, by a planned diet and a lot of exercise, he attained the desired goal. More remarkably, he lost about 22 kg of fat and simultaneously gained 5 kg of muscle mass. The net effect was about 17 kg weight loss. We will discuss Aamir Khan's weight loss journey in detail in subsequent chapters.

How Do I Know This?

Now, you may have picked up this book because the cover says Aamir Khan has written the foreword. While his story is amazing, you may wonder who am I to be telling you these things? Let me start by saying, the book you are reading is nearly thirty-five years in the making. This is the length of my career in obesity which started on 5 February 1983, when I joined my father at his clinics at Charni Road in Mumbai. Sure, I was a doctor and could treat patients for most things, but I was not familiar with treating obesity. They don't teach that in the medical school. Therefore, my first several months were spent sitting silently next to him, watching as he worked with patients, taking case notes. When I first started seeing patients for myself, my father would sometimes take the day off. On days when he was not in the clinic, much to my disappointment, some patients who had appointments would peek into the clinic and on seeing me sitting at the desk alone would say, 'Oh, *toh Bade Doctor Sahib aaj nahin hain*? (Oh, the senior doctor is not in today?)' They would then quickly leave the exam room and mutter to the secretary, '*Main kal aunga* (I will come tomorrow).'

Of course, after some time I learned well from my father. Patients started trusting me, and seeing results. We continued the practice together quite successfully. When I felt I was ready to branch out, I opened an additional obesity clinic in 1985 at Ghatkopar, Mumbai. All along, my passion was obesity treatment. It was tremendously gratifying to help patients. But there was always a nagging itch at the back of my mind. Medical schools then, and even now, do not do a good job of providing training in nutrition. I needed all the training I could get to handle a nutrition-related condition with authority. I took one year off from my obesity practice and went to the US to obtain a Master of Science degree in nutrition. Those were some crazy times. As a graduate student, I managed jobs as a teaching assistant and a research assistant and working day and night, completed a two-year course of classes and research in eleven months. As I returned to India and rejoined my obesity practice, I focused on helping the obese patient in front of me. But as 100 patients turned into 1,000 patients, and 1,000 turned into 1,000 new patients every year, I gained a different perspective on obesity. It was clearly a disease and not just a cosmetic issue. Otherwise, it would be an easy fix. The deeper, unanswered question hanging over everything was why do so many people need help? My pursuit of an answer to this question brought me to America for the next twenty-five years.

During the course of my MS, I got a taste of research and science. Medicine is driven by science. As a doctor, I employed the discoveries made by science. But here I saw a whole new world of scientists making the discoveries that I would use in my practice. It was exhilarating to see 'behind the curtain'. This experience made me realize that the question – why do people suffer obesity – was still unanswered. I decided that I wanted to find the answer to this. I joined the famed University Department of Chemical Technology, of the University of Bombay, for a PhD programme in biochemistry, while I continued my practice. You can imagine the workload. Due to the pressure of medical school education, I got into the habit of sleeping only three to four hours at night. This new life was no different.

Till date, I joke that my wife would not recognize me if I ever came home from work in broad daylight.

During my PhD studies, a chance conversation with Professor S.M. Ajinkya, a family friend, renowned veterinary pathologist and one-time dean of Bombay Veterinary College, completely transformed my life and led to the development of a new field of research in obesity known as Infectobesity, or 'Obesity of Infectious Origin'. One afternoon, over a cup of tea in his home, Dr Ajinkya described his research on SMAM-1, a virus that he had discovered – and therefore bore his initials. He explained the symptoms of this viral infection caused in chickens. Chickens infected with SMAM-1 have big and pale livers, big kidneys, a lot of fat in the abdomen and their other organs. He kept talking, but for me, everything else switched off.

'Fat in the abdomen…did he say fat in the abdomen?' My mind latched on to those words. Why was there a lot of fat in the abdomen of chickens infected with SMAM-1? Is the virus making these chickens fat? I could hear myself asking these questions to myself, and then to Dr Ajinkya. He stopped drinking tea and looked at me with his signature kind, caring yet thoughtful smile, and said, 'I don't know.' These three important words changed my world (and I believe later changed the world to some extent as well). He could have said, 'I don't think that SMAM-1 increases fat in chickens,' and I would have believed him and moved on. But he was an open-minded scientist, trained to say the truth as-is. If you don't know, simply say so. He then added, 'You are working on a PhD, why don't you find this answer by actually conducting experiments with SMAM-1 in chickens?'

I already had a lot of research studies planned for my PhD. Now, I added one more. You can imagine the scepticism around this concept in the late 1980s. With few available resources, we conducted our first experiment. Guess what? The chickens that were infected with SMAM-1 and the chickens that were kept in the cages of these infected chickens became very fat compared to uninfected control chickens that were maintained in a separate room. It was particularly interesting to see the chickens that shared cages with infected chickens also developed obesity. This meant that the infected chickens passed on the infection as well as obesity to their cage mates. So, could obesity spread? It was a scary thought. I remember that day like it was just yesterday. I don't know how I made it home, or if I ate anything at all. All I remember is the unbelievable excitement and fear. Excitement at the new discovery, for the first time in the world to show that a chicken virus can cause obesity, and fear about the validity of our research. Was this true? Was it possible that a viral infection could cause obesity? If yes, why had no one in the world reported it by now? I wondered if I was really this fortunate to step into such an important discovery this early in my life, at the age of twenty-nine?

Fortunately, science has a solution to address these fears. It is called replication. We painstakingly repeated the same experiment with more number of chickens and obtained the same results. Now, I was losing fear, gaining confidence but also becoming anxious. Anxious about how I could further this discovery to ultimately help people with obesity. Our experiment with humans was the final straw. My next study showed that 20 per cent of the people coming to my clinic for obesity treatment whom we examined were exposed to SMAM-1 infection in the past, and these people were heavier than those without such infection. Perhaps, these people were probably exposed to SMAM-1 while handling chickens or eggs that were infected with the virus. That was just a guess. At this point, I realized that we were onto an important discovery. The possibilities of something beneficial resulting from this research for people affected with obesity were very real. But there was a problem. The research facilities available in the US were not the same that we had in India back then.

My only solution was to close my practice in India and move back to USA to conduct this research. It was not an easy decision. As a matter of fact, I was likely one of the top obesity practitioners in India at the time. There were umpteen reasons to not take this drastic step. Too many relatives, friends and well-wishers pointed at the cushy life we had in Mumbai and alerted us to the financially disastrous implications if we left. After some serious thought, I shut down my three clinics, and my wife, our son and I packed our belongings in six suitcases and took a big leap of faith to the United States.

I had accepted a research job in the US. It meant a 95 per cent pay cut. The job was not in the field of obesity. We had given ourselves two years to find a research job that would let me work in virus-induced obesity, failing which, we were to return to Mumbai. We did not wish to live in a foreign land if I was not going to pursue research of my dreams. After two years of constant trying, hopes and disappointments, and a life below the poverty line, there was no job in obesity research. The US was experiencing a bad economic situation in the early 1990s. Our self-imposed, two-year deadline approached and we decided to return to India. With a turn of events fit for a movie plot, a month before our return, I got a nice research job in the department of medicine at the University of Wisconsin. The persistence finally paid off. At the University of Wisconsin, we discovered another virus – Ad36, a human virus that causes obesity. Initially, many researchers found it hard to believe our pioneering research. In conferences, after my talk on the topic, I would get audience responses that ranged from 'preposterous' to 'Nobel Prize winning' work. I would remember the story of Badshah and Birbal ki Khichdi, where a person wins a big prize by standing overnight in the freezing water of a lake and spends that time by looking at distant city lights. I kept going in the hope that it will all change one day. Our data were too strong, and I had confidence in our science.

A modern-day real story helped me stay on my path. This is the story of two Australian scientists, Drs Marshall and Warren, who discovered that stomach ulcers are caused by bacteria. Until then, the world believed that spicy food, stress and anxiety caused ulcers. In fact, in medical school, we learnt that stomach ulcers are caused by hurry, worry and curry! Their discovery was so radical that not many people believed the findings for a number of years. One day, Dr Marshall decided to end this disbelief of people in their findings. He drank the solution containing *Helicobacter pylori*, the bacteria that cause ulcers, and proved to the world once and for all that bacteria cause ulcers. Opinions changed rapidly after this dramatic move and now, the antibiotic treatment for getting rid of these bacteria is a standard treatment for ulcers. Drs Warren and Marshall won the Nobel Prize in 2005 for their discovery.

Numerous studies from our group, and many other groups from around the world, have now firmly established the role of infections in obesity, and Infectobesity, a term I coined, has widespread usage. This research is important as it may be possible to develop a vaccine to prevent one type of obesity due to infections. Another, more significant reason, is that while there are also other examples, the fact that infections could cause obesity clearly shows that obesity is a disease and not simply a choice, or failure of will power. You may literally be 'catching' obesity. Over the years, TV, radio, Internet and other magazines have shown a lot of interest in our research. Many documentaries are made on this topic, including one by the National Geographic titled

Fat Plague, which depicts my life and research. All this has truly helped in getting the word out to people suffering from obesity. Over the years, I have received numerous emails, letters and in-person messages, simply thanking me (which should deservedly go to our research team as well) for making the point that there can be causes of obesity that are outside the control of a person.

When we first discovered that SMAM-1 causes obesity, I was thinking if that was just one lucky chance and whether I will ever discover anything this important again. Now, I know that we discovered another virus, Ad36, which causes obesity. These discoveries led other world researchers to discover additional similar viruses that cause obesity. Moreover, we are currently developing a powerful drug against diabetes that is made from a virus. It turns out that this series of scientific success stories is not a one-time lucky chance.

Well, you can see what has shaped this book. My education, research training, years of experience from obesity practice and research, including success and frustration, have all shaped my thoughts. It has taken thirty-five years to create this book, because it has taken me thirty-five years to learn obesity from root to fruit. I have seen the evolution of science behind the treatment. I have seen and fought against quackery and self-serving misleading nutrition themes that keep mushrooming. When you read this book, know that what you are reading is the unvarnished truth. I wish to reach out to people beyond just those whom I individually interact with. I wish to reach out to you, the reader, to help find a way through the maze of diets in front of you. It is my pleasure and honour to do so.

Picking Your Way Through the Diet Book Maze

There are many opinions out there about how to lose fat. Several diet books are cropping up, promising the best results. While some of these opinions are useful, many are not. As a nutrition researcher, I have been trained to say only what is scientific. And, I instil the same onto the minds of my students and trainees. I dare not say or write anything that is unscientific, lest my scientist colleagues, whom I respect so much, eat me up with their criticism. My reputation in their eyes is important to me. More importantly, I owe it to my patients and to readers to inform with facts about nutrition. So, being careful about scientific or clinical validity of statements has become my second nature (as it is to any good researcher).

With this background, it pains me to see how so many diet books have a casual relationship with scientific truth. While reading these books, I would get stuck on every page. Wait. Why did you say that? Where is the evidence? Did you not just make it up? I would think. Then, I started seeing a common pattern in these books that freely bend truth. The books could profess very different theories for weight loss, but they were similar in using two strategies. The first strategy I call 'A fast one'. I can best describe this approach by sharing with you an example of a pitch I once heard on a CD. It said something like this, 'Are you tired when you wake up? Do you feel overwhelmed with the work you have? Is there too much stress in your life? Do you think you really need a break? Are you really really tired at the end of the day? If yes, then the blue-green algae from volcanic lakes is perfect for you.' Get the strategy? There are so many statements that you are almost guaranteed to experience. Who does not feel tired at the end of the day? Who does not want a vacation? And, they are also counting on you agreeing with them. Many are likely to be amazed about how they understood your condition. And, when you are in such agreeable mood, they slide their 'fast one'. They say that the blue-green algae is perfect for you, and you agree. Where is the connection between you feeling tired and the blue-green algae? How does your feeling stressed make blue-green algae good for you? You will notice a similar approach in many diet books. They will tell you what you already know – that you have excess weight, that you are not in best of health physically or mentally, that your social interaction may be suffering, that you don't feel energetic, that you are having late nights and too much stress. You agree. And, then they advance their favourite theory, which you accept. You are sold.

This is followed by the second trick, which I call 'smoke and mirrors'. Think about this: If I give you a weight loss diet plan that says eat a certain type of breakfast, lunch, evening snack and a dinner. This could be effective but not attractive for you. You may not see anything special in these instructions. The solution? I make up theories and practices for you that are completely baseless but sound like major rituals. For example, instead of the mundane (but scientific and effective) advice, I will make up restrictions for you: don't eat white coloured food in mornings, don't drink tea between 4 and 6 p.m., eat only with left leg touching the ground while facing the East, or whatever. You get the idea.

A variation of this trick is to make sure you are eating less, which is the real reason for losing weight, but to credit your weight loss to something different. An example is the HCG programme. Human Chorionic Gonadotropin (HCG) is a hormone mainly secreted from the placenta, the part that attaches a baby to mother in uterus. Injections of this expensive hormone are touted to produce weight loss. Real deal? You are also asked to have a very low calorie diet, which is what making you lose weight. Interestingly, to catch attention, such programmes are marketed as 'lose weight without diet'. Once, a patient came in with her brother. 'I don't believe in dieting for losing weight', the brother declared. I continued counseling my patient, not wanting to take the brother's bait and waste time. 'I am following a programme to lose weight without diet. You have to take cold-water showers three times a day. That's it.'. He persisted. 'And of course, eat sensibly and less etc....' He said. See the clever plan here? Eat less is what reduces weight, but taking showers gets credit.

Why this book?

Please read this sentence carefully: Obesity is a serious and complex disease with multiple causes, but with few effective, meaningful and lasting treatment options. Dr Albert Stunkard, a famous obesity researcher said, 'Most people with obesity will not enter treatment programmes, of those who do take treatment, most will not lose weight and of those who do lose weight, most will regain it.' The sad part is that this was written in 1958, and even after worldwide intense research in the field, the sentence still holds true. Yet, many diet books seem to make light of the serious disease, or not recognize efforts that obesity treatment requires. Some books emphasize your looks. How you can look better if you lose weight and how you can get the body of movie stars. The doctor in me thinks this is misleading. Have you heard of any doctor advocating the treatment of cancer so you could look better? Treat diabetes to look like a star? If not, then why is the disease of obesity an exception? It is possible that some wish to focus on weight loss to look better. But, it is the job of an expert to draw attention of those people to the physical and mental health benefits of weight loss, not keep discussing how different you would look with weight loss.

In our obesity clinic, especially in the United States, I have often been asked questions about the body size of our staff. We employ staff of all body sizes. If patients were treated by a slim staff member, I would hear that, 'These thin people couldn't possibly understand the struggles of a person with obesity.' On the other hand, if the staff member was a larger person, the complaint would be, 'Look at this person, if a member of their own team is huge, how will I ever lose weight?' Sounds like a no-win situation. But the answer is simple. Obesity is a disease. Check out the declaration to that effect by the American Medical Association, the Obesity Society and similar highly respected organizations. You don't catch obesity. Obesity catches you. Some people are affected with it while some others are not. Some struggle lifelong to manage weight and some can do it easily. Expecting that staff of obesity clinic to be free from human diseases such as obesity is akin to expecting all cardiologists to be free from heart disease. It is too vain to brag about your body or body shape, if you don't have the disease obesity. But, you will read more about this later.

Another jaw-dropping ignorance sometimes propagated in popular media is a complete unfamiliarity with medical facts about the processes of digestion and metabolism. Digestion is a process that starts in our mouth when we eat food and continues through the stomach and intestines. During this process, food is broken down into smaller components that are then absorbed in the body from the intestinal walls. If digestion is improper or inadequate, food does not break down into these components and is thus not absorbed. It is excreted in the form of faeces. Now, compare this medical fact with what you may have come across. How many times have you heard that eating certain things, impairs your digestion, which results in body fat deposition? Quite the contrary. If your digestion is impaired, you are less likely to gain calories from food and less likely to store fat. In fact, orlistat, a legitimate drug available for obesity, does just that. It interferes with fat digestion. So, of the total fat you eat, about one-third does not get digested and gets thrown out in stools. Thus, your body gets fewer calories from food and you lose weight. Armed with this information, feel free to question the next time you hear how poor digestion can lead to more body fat.

Traditionally, not recognizing that obesity is a serious medical condition has left its treatment mainly in the hands of well-meaning friends and family and ill-meaning quacks. As a result, we have not seen the same aggressive push for developing effective obesity treatments, that some other chronic diseases experience. It is little wonder then that we have not seen better success in obesity management in the past sixty years.

Now, here is something very important. Although we certainly need better and more effective treatments for fat loss, we do have treatment approaches that have worked for numerous people in India and across the world. However, too many false promises and fake treatments have crowded out the legitimate treatment approaches to the extent that people cannot tell them apart. This book is an effort to convey that it is indeed possible to successfully lose fat and exactly how it can be done.

A lifestyle change that includes physical activity and a well-designed diet plan can improve health and help with fat loss. However, all diets are not designed to be the same. Some diets recommend that you simply change your overall lifestyle, push yourself away from the table, eat less, exercise more, make a few changes to your life. That's it? Is this Band-Aid going to tackle a serious disease such as obesity? I understand that it is hard for people to tell the difference between nutrition facts vs fiction. It is up to those who have really studied nutrition science, to set the record straight. This book is my attempt.

Some theories condemn most currently available foods and encourage us to simply go back to our diet from the past. Sure, a lifestyle change and careful consumption of food is beneficial to us as an increasingly consumerist society but these changes may not always work for someone suffering from obesity. You may have heard that the way our ancestors consumed food was the best way and it is something you should emulate. This implies that the diet from the Palaeolithic Stone Age is the best. Pause and think – why? Why is that diet better than today's? The average life span during the Stone Age was thought to be twenty-eight years and it is well above seventy today in many countries, especially in the countries we love bashing for their present-day diets. Clear evidence from unearthed skeletons has shown the terrible state of dental health of Egyptians during the pyramid-building times. It is attributed to their diet. Just about sixty years ago, life expectancy in India was near forty years, which is now about sixty-eight years. I suppose you realize where I am going with this. Numerous factors may influence our health, including the diet.

It is hard to justify abandoning a diet associated with a time of greater health and life expectancy, in favour of a diet from a period of poor life expectancy. Moreover, the dietary approaches need to be realistic and practical. Humans have toiled too much to innovate present-day comforts. We are not stopping the use of microwaves, readymade products or cars, and we are not going back to chopping trees for cooking meals or running after animals for food. This is the reality and we need to accept it. This book does not advocate extreme diets that require you to change everything about how you live and force you to trade leanness for happiness. Modern day nutrition science has shown us how to pick good things from many cultures, many countries and use them creatively. The traditional Indian diet is no exception, it is full of great benefits. The trick is to combine such nutrition health tips from global cultures and design strategic diets that make it possible to lose and maintain weight, with the least possible disruption to your life and lifestyle because this is the type of diet you are likely to follow for a long time.

I believe in scientific fat loss, using methods that have been tested and re-tested and proven to work. If you believe in this as well, this book may be the answer for you. This book does not claim that fat loss is easy or that you could lose hundreds of kilos of fat without much effort. It does not blame or shame you for having excess fat, or for having tried and failed in the past. I know the disease of obesity up close and I know the struggle of people who are affected by it. This book will first explain the scientific facts around obesity. Next, it will help you address your biology, such that the body will resist less when you are trying to lose weight. It will help you navigate social and cultural situations that can ruin any diet, in a way that maintains social relationships. And finally, the book will help you manage your innate drive to eat or crave food. By the end of it, you should have a good perspective on what it takes to lose fat and keep it off, with a diet that is practical and possible.

My book is for both adult men and women. It is not about building muscle but is certainly about maximizing fat loss and minimizing muscle loss. It also provides instructions that are gender specific and consider the differences in male and female bodies. On a lighter note, perhaps, I should warn readers about a potential side effect. I experienced this on three separate occasions. Substantial loss of fat had brought about dramatic transformation in these women, including a great boost to their confidence and the ability and willingness to interact socially. Apparently, this was unsettling for their respective husbands, who tried to sabotage their efforts in many ways. It is truly astonishing that these husbands were jealous and worried about the achievements of their respective wives. I must admit, I can help you with obesity, but I do not know how to prevent such a response from your spouse to your success. There, you are on your own!

2

Protein Power: A Secret to Losing Weight and Keeping It Off

B aton Rouge, Louisiana, USA, is known for its incredible food, the best live music you will hear outside New Orleans and friendly locals. When I was a professor living here, I used to take frequent walks around a lake near the University. Its placid waters reflected the colours of breathtaking Louisiana sunrises and sunsets. Lakeside property is as gorgeous as it is expensive and has only one drawback – every once in a while, someone will find in their garden a two-metre alligator that has crawled out from the lake.

I had two close friends here. Let's call them George and Shrikant. George was a physically and mentally fit, retired mechanical engineer in his early seventies. Shrikant was in his mid-fifties; an NRI lawyer from Delhi. The three of us were weekend walkers who enjoyed discussions, debates and arguments during our walks. The duration of our walk depended on the intensity of the discussion. The more debatable a topic, the longer the walk. One Saturday morning, at the start of our walk, George fired the opening shot, 'Nikhil, nine out of ten Indians don't get enough protein. Did you know that?' Shrikant said, 'Wait, how do you know this?' George pulled out his phone and showed us a headline in the *Times of India*. I had seen the story before.

It was not surprising that George had picked up on an article with the word 'protein' in it. This was his favourite nutrition word. He was a college-level football champion, and his knowledge of nutrition was based on what his coaches had told him in the 1960s. He often proclaimed that he was a 'pure non-vegetarian', meaning he had never eaten anything other than fish, meat, chicken, eggs or milk. No bread, no fruits, no vegetables. Ever. He joked that he loved fruits and vegetables too dearly to eat them. In fact, during my obesity practice in India, I had come across only two such patients with the exact same dietary preference.

George continued, 'Why don't Indians eat protein?'

Shrikant chimed in, 'We eat plenty of protein. Just because we don't eat bacon and steak for breakfast, lunch and dinner doesn't mean we don't eat protein.'

'That's not what this article says. And you say there's so much obesity in India. How do they gain weight eating just those fruits and vegetables?'

Shrikant said, 'George, your ignorance shines through again. The only reason that these numbers are so low is because majority of Indians are impoverished, with no access to protein-rich foods.'

'Okay,' I said, 'you're both right and wrong. Protein is really important, but, you know, there are other important nutrients too'.

'Of course, I know,' George responded, 'vitamins and minerals. I take a multivitamin tablet every day.'

I knew they needed a quick lesson in the basic concepts of nutrition, so I explained: 'Besides protein, vitamins and minerals, other key components of the food we eat are carbohydrates, fat, alcohol, fibre and water. Sugar is an example of carbohydrate, egg white is a protein, and cooking oil, butter or ghee as they use in India are examples of fat. Most foods have carbohydrates, protein and fat in varying proportions. And, even if you intend to eat only proteins, you are often eating these other components. Wheat, rice or noodles have all three, protein, carbs and fat, as does milk. Meat has protein and fat. Fruits and vegetables have carbohydrates, vitamins, minerals and fibre. Fibre is the indigestible part of food that has lot of health benefits.'

'See?' Shrikant interjected, 'protein isn't everything, George. We're not alligators. People can survive without it.'

'Er, not really, Shrikant,' I said. 'Protein is actually a critical nutrient.' Almost everything in the body, from skin to organs, to blood, nerves are made from the proteins we eat. Our body can manufacture fat or carbohydrates (sugars) by converting protein. However, the opposite does not happen. Sugars or fats in diet cannot be turned into proteins. Therefore, the body is entirely dependent for protein from the food we eat. Denying proteins to body, for whatever reason, can have serious consequences.

'Carbohydrates, or sugars, starches, carbs, or glucose as we call them are the energy source for cells of our body. Carbohydrates from foods such as rice, bread or potato are broken down by digestion into individual units called glucose. Cells in our body, including brain cells, use this glucose to produce energy. Carbohydrates are so essential for survival, that if carbohydrates are in short supply, body breaks down muscle, or uses protein from food to convert it to glucose for energy. Bottom line: to give protein to your body, you have no choice but to eat protein-containing food.'

I stopped to take a breath under one of the 200-year-old oak trees that surround the lake and the university. But George persisted, 'So Indians don't like proteins? Is that why they don't eat proteins?'

'Could it be,' said Shrikant, 'that protein is expensive? Nikhil, all the foods you described – meat, milk, etc., – are expensive in India.'

I said, 'Yes, it's true that good sources of proteins are costlier in India, and economic conditions force individuals to eat lesser proteins. But surprisingly, lower protein intake is also seen in well-to-do families in India.'

They were both shocked by that, but if you think it through, it will make sense. I explained that protein is, indeed, by far the most neglected component in Indian nutrition. Good sources of protein in Indian diet are eggs, meat, chicken, fish, milk, soybean, pulses or daal, nuts and, to some extent, wheat. Now, consider our traditional customs and culture around diet. Even those who are non-vegetarians tend to exclude non-vegetarian food several days in a week for religious reasons. Some are even stricter, and in addition to non-vegetarian food, avoid foods such as daal, or lentil and wheat on many days of the week for religious reasons. Somehow, protein-containing foods, barring milk, take a backseat on many days of the month.

'I had never thought of it that way,' said Shrikant.

'Right, Shrikant,' I said, 'think about this, too. When you hear the word "wholesome", which foods come to mind? What are the foods that we tell pregnant women or a new mother to eat for health?'

Shrikant thought for a minute and said, 'Ghee. Sugar. And milk.'

'Exactly,' I said, 'these are all praised as energy-giving foods. Not protein. Protein is not recognized as wholesome. Now, this is not a negative commentary on our cultural practices. Rather, it is an honest attempt to recognize the state of nutrition. Most of my patients are *not* poor or undernourished. On the contrary, their chief struggle is *excess* weight. However, probably because common dietary practices in India undervalue the role of foods containing protein, they generally get less protein in their diet.'

'It's possible,' I said, 'that this lower protein intake by Indians is contributing to their weight gain.'

'I don't buy it,' said Shrikant, 'I know fat's worse for you. You told me that once. Fat has more calories than protein.'

'Correct,' I said, '1 gram of protein has 4 calories, 1 gram of carbohydrates has 4 calories, and 1 gram of fat has 9 calories.'

'Bingo,' said Shrikant.

George asked, 'I like the sound of it. Protein is important. But, why would protein be responsible for weight gain in Indians?'

The answer to that question rests in what is called the Protein Leverage Hypothesis. This is an intriguing theory based on animal and human studies. Based on this theory, protein is so essential for the body's survival that humans are driven to acquire a specific amount of protein each day through food. In some ways, our tongue and body sifts through the food we eat to determine if we have eaten enough amount of protein for the day. If the food you eat has insufficient protein, the body prompts you to feel hungry and go seek some more food to meet your protein quota.

How does this lead to weight gain? A diet that is poor in protein will drive you to eat more food in the hope of getting protein, which gives additional calories, which leads to fat gain. There are human studies that tested low, medium and higher protein amount in diet and monitored the food intake of these study participants for days. It was observed that those eating lower protein in their food felt hungrier and unknowingly ended up consuming significantly more calories. As per the theory, their bodies simply sensed that their food had lower protein and decided to make them eat more.

As per these studies, for a person who requires 2,000 calories in a day, 50g of proteins would be considered low intake, 75g would be considered medium and 125g would be considered high protein intake. Now, compare this with the current protein intake of Indians. According to a recent report by the Federation of Indian Chambers of Commerce and Industry (FICCI)[1], daily protein consumption at the national level dipped from 60.2g for a person in 1993–94 to 56.5g in 2011–12 in rural areas and from 57.2g to 55.7g in urban areas. This data reveals several interesting points. First, on an average, the amount of protein that Indians consume is at a level that is likely to promote more hunger and more eating. Second, our protein intake has fallen in the last twenty years, exactly when rates of obesity increased. We don't know with certainty whether or not this is the only contributing factor to increased obesity. There could be other contributors as well. However, it makes you stop and think. The same FICCI report also mentioned that as Indians decreased their protein intake, the consumption of fats and oils increased by 25–30 per cent. Perhaps, as a nation, the lower protein intake is making us hungrier, driving us to eat more fatty food, that has double the calories, leading to weight gain.

'Amazing!' George exclaimed. 'So interesting that different countries may have different reasons for weight gain. I suppose

---

1 https://timesofindia.indiatimes.com/india/Protein-intake-in-India-dips-10-oil-fat-consumption-up/articleshow/47169586.cms

they need different ways to lose weight.' Shrikant said, 'Yes, take it from me. I need an Indian diet. How convenient we have Nikhil here.'

As we neared the end of our now about 10 km walk, George said, 'Well, Nikhil, you've got me. Sounds like I've got to stick to my pure non-vegetarian diet. It's good for me.' Just then I noticed a straight ripple crossed the surface, probably an alligator underneath. Shrikant pointed at it and said, 'George, you meat-eater, you must have been an alligator in a past life.'

'Or the next one,' George replied.

The Best Bread in Brazil

Out of every country I have visited, including the European countries, I have never tasted better bread than I have in Brazil. Sorry, France. Also, I found Brazilian cuisine quite like Indian cuisine. Spices, flavours and even the variety of food were familiar to my Indian palette. Pink guava, that we ate only sometimes during my childhood, was my favourite fruit while in Brazil.

The chance to try amazing Brazilian bread presented itself when I was invited to give a talk at the International Congress on Obesity (ICO). I was to lecture about our research regarding obesity caused by viral infections. The ICO was organized by the International Association for the Study of Obesity, an umbrella organization of national obesity societies worldwide. Many scientists who are internationally known for their contribution attend the conference. It is always such a remarkable experience for me to meet these luminary researchers. My Indian mind thinks of them as 'rishis' and 'maharshis' described in Indian mythologies, who are engrossed in pursuit of knowledge in their ashram-like laboratories. These researchers are incredibly passionate about their field. Many of them have spent their entire lives in research, discovering science to help those suffering from obesity. Try talking with them about weather or politics. They will quickly bring you back to talking about their research, or yours.

One such person is Dr Anoop Misra, an obesity researcher from New Delhi. I met him for the first time in Brazil. He had given a great presentation on why Indians should be considered 'obese' at a weight lower than that used for defining obesity in the western world. Dr Misra and other research groups have discovered a peculiarity of a typical Indian body, compared to Caucasians from the US or the United Kingdom. They observed that if you compare two individuals of same body weight, one Indian, and the other Caucasian, the Indian person will have less muscle mass and more body fat compared to the Caucasian. Due to the greater body fat, the Indian man or woman typically faces greater obesity-related health risk such as diabetes or heart disease.

Another disadvantage for Indians is our lower muscle mass. One in every five to six Indians over sixty-five years of age has very low muscle mass[2]. Our muscles largely determine the calorie need for the day. Smaller muscles mean less calorie burning, which makes weight gain that much easier, and harder to lose.[3] It is also linked with additional health issues such as inadequate response to our hormones such as insulin, making it easier for blood glucose levels to increase. Researchers have known for a long time that any time you lose weight, it is fat and muscle. It's hard to lose only fat without losing some muscle. Now you can see the dual disadvantage that we Indians face. As it is, we have relatively lower muscle mass. On top of it, if we lose a lot of muscle during weight loss, we simply make it easier to gain that weight back. If we have less muscle mass to begin with, it's important to preserve what we have. This also applies to women, who don't strive for building muscles like a body builder. Nonetheless, humans need muscles to function, to move, sit, walk, run and more. Losing muscle unnecessarily can have similar consequences for women as well.

With all this doom and gloom, it might seem our case is hopeless. Indeed, much is stacked against the Indian who seeks to lose weight. But do not despair. A solution exists – a solution to minimize how much muscle you lose during weight loss. This is, in fact, a very important aspect of successful weight management. It can separate a run-of-the-

---

2   https://www.ncbi.nlm.nih.gov/pmc/articles/PMC4864288/
3   https://www.ncbi.nlm.nih.gov/pmc/articles/PMC2633408/

mill weight management programme from a really effective one. The secret to this solution is a technique that I call Protein Power.

What is Protein Power?

There are three key reasons to pay special attention to proteins when you are trying to lose weight.

Protein Power can be cleverly used to:

- Reduce hunger and feel full during dieting
- Increase fat loss
- Prevent weight regain

If you have tried losing weight, you certainly don't want to be miserably hungry. You want to lose fat quickly and you want to keep it off permanently. Is it possible? Yes. It is possible to develop your diet plan in such a way that will strategically reduce hunger, minimize loss of muscle protein and promote loss of fat and reduce weight regain. And, proteins play a big role in such a plan. In subsequent chapters, we are going to see how to put this to work in a practical way. Here's how you can use protein smartly to your benefit:

Reduce hunger and feel full: Over the past sixteen years, my group of researchers conducted several studies to discover that eggs have the wonderful property of making you feel full and keeping you feeling that way for a long time. Eggs are the source of the highest quality proteins. In research participants, we compared the effects of breakfast containing eggs to another breakfast without eggs, but of equivalent calories and weight. It turns out, this simple trick of eating eggs for breakfast kept people full for a long time and they ate less during the lunch that followed. Moreover, when we had study participants on weight-loss diets, those who ate eggs lost weight faster. If the participants were not on a weight-loss diet, just eating eggs made no difference to their weight. The message: If you eat high quality protein such as whole eggs, it keeps you feeling full and that lets you stick to your diet without temptation or cheating and thus speeds up weight loss. Before you start loading your plate with eggs, remember that eggs don't work their magic if you are not on a weight-loss diet. They only *supplement* your weight-loss efforts, not replace them.

Increase fat loss: As we discussed earlier, while dieting, our goal is to minimize the loss of muscle and increase fat loss. This is possible by adding protein to your diet. One research study[4] showed that when people lost weight, about one-third of it was loss of muscle. However, this percentage is much less for those who ate higher amount of protein during weight

---

4   https://www.ncbi.nlm.nih.gov/pubmed/18589032

loss. Another study demonstrated this very nicely.[5] In this, groups of participants were started on a weight-loss diet, and the groups were given diets that contained increasing amounts of proteins. With higher protein intake, participants lost more weight and less muscle. The message: it is not enough to just count calories in a weight-loss diet. The diet also needs to include higher protein amounts.

Prevent weight regain: This is my favourite and I bet it will become your favourite too. Those of you have tried losing weight already know how disheartening it is to see all that lost weight come back slowly, but surely. I am often reminded of a quote by Mark Twain about quitting smoking. He said, 'Giving up smoking is real easy. I have done it hundreds of times.' Similarly, many people have lost hundreds of kilograms of weight, if you add up all their attempts. Reality is, and you may not hear this truth from too many people, that if you have the tendency to gain weight, it is hard to totally stop that weight regain. Your body will continue to take you back to your original weight. Nonetheless, it is possible to offer stiff opposition and slow down the process of regain. Retaining your muscle mass while losing weight is the key. Better muscle mass helps you burn more calories and reduces the risk of weight regain. The message: All weight losses are not equal.

---

5   https://www.ncbi.nlm.nih.gov/pmc/articles/PMC3159052/

A systematic weight loss achieved by eating good amount of protein will go a long way in reducing weight regain.

If you are reading about Protein Power for the first time, it is likely that you are excited about these many wonderful properties of protein. I know such excitement first hand. But, slow down. When I was nineteen years old, I read a book about Pritikin's Diet. It extolled the virtues of fruits, vegetables and fibre. The book said foods containing fibre were good for you. I was reading this for the first time and I was sold. Eager to change my lifestyle and diet, I wanted to eat more fibre from fruits. That night, we had pomegranate in the house. Normally, I would just chew on those pinkish-red seeds and spit them out. But, I was all pumped up to eat more fibre! Seeds have more fibre, I reasoned. I ate the entire pomegranate, seed and skin and all. I spent the entire night rolling in pain due to stomach ache. I learned my lesson about moderation. Some fibre is good for you. That does not mean a lot more would be better.

The same concept can be extended to protein intake. Protein is good but excessive protein, considered as a 'high protein diet', may not be the best thing for everyone. It may not be safe or healthy for all. Eating too much protein for a long time can put a load on the liver and kidneys, the two key organs that handle protein digestion. Some concerns have been expressed about the safety of a diet high in protein. I would rather not test the safety of a diet on any of you. I do not recommend a very high protein diet that includes 150–200g protein a day. To get this much protein, one would have to eat about 22–28 eggs per day, or drink 18–25 glasses of milk. Instead, a diet only moderately high in protein can achieve best results without the safety concerns. This sweet spot is somewhere between 70–110g of protein per day and depends on individual's body weight, as we will see.

I've received several emails, like the one below, regarding excessive protein intake.

> 'Dear Doctor, I am very thin and wish to build my body and gain muscle like Mr Aamir Khan. I have been taking protein supplements twice a day for the past six months. Why have I not gained muscle even though I am eating so much protein?'

If you have a similar question in mind, read on. There is nothing wrong in aspiring to have a muscular body. However, many people misunderstand Protein Power. Proteins, or protein supplements, do not automatically help you build muscle. You must also exercise appropriately. More muscle building needs more exercise. When you exercise adequately, the body tries to build new muscle. In such a situation, proteins in food or supplements can provide that extra raw material to aid this process. Without exercise, all that extra protein could simply get converted to fat and get stored in the body.

We researchers have a habit, we think about our research almost non-stop. The famous philosopher Henry David Thoreau said, 'This world is a canvas to our imagination.' Similarly, we researchers are mesmerized by the world around us and feel like kids in a candy store. New ideas for research keep popping like germinating seeds. It is so tempting to test them all. The only thing that keeps us from testing all these ideas is reality. The reality that we have only so much time, money and resources to conduct research. This hard reality keeps us in check and we prioritize. We test only the most promising ideas. While conducting our studies with proteins and weight loss, I had such a thought, 'If eating too much high protein is not good for your health, could we use high *quality* of protein, instead of *quantity*, and get better benefits without having to eat large quantity?' By the way, the quality of protein is determined based on how that protein rates in its effect on growth. Generally, proteins from animal sources such as the egg protein, meat, chicken, fish, milk are considered to have higher quality, and proteins of vegetable origin, such as beans and pulses have relatively lower quality. So, could quality be a substitute for quantity in this case? Would eating smaller amounts of high quality protein food such as eggs be as effective in increasing fullness than eating greater quantity protein from a bread or roti, which has lower quality protein? This research is in progress.

Meanwhile, a series of studies were recently published that compared various non-vegetarian foods such as beef and beans or beef and soybean tofu. The results were interesting.

Whether you ate beef or a vegetarian protein source, that had little to no effect on hunger or food intake. This is especially good news for Indian vegetarians, who cannot or will not eat non-vegetarian food. No problem. Research indicates that eating an adequate amount of vegetarian sources of protein can pack same the punch against hunger.

Let's bust another popular myth about protein quality. Have you heard that eating raw food is the best diet for weight loss? This claim is not limited to eating raw fruits or vegetables, but also includes eating raw wheat, rice, beans, pulses, etc. The theory is that foods are nutritionally better if eaten raw, and that is how mother nature intended they be consumed. Well, it's true that certain vitamins such as vitamins B or C are lost to some extent in cooking, but there are many major problems with theory.

Problem 1: It is a scientific fact that the nutritional quality of many foods, especially those containing proteins is vastly improved by cooking them. Cooking makes proteins undergo a process called denaturation, which makes them easy to digest and easy for our body to use them. The same is true for many other nutrients. Carbohydrates from rice or wheat are much more available for the body, when cooked, than when in raw form.

Problem 2: It is argued that this raw diet is more nutritious because our ancestors ate raw food. Not true. In fact, when humans were evolving from small apes to modern-day humans, you notice a sudden change in the skeleton sizes of prehistoric ancestors. Some time they stopped being small monkey-like creatures and started looking more like modern day humans. Their skull size and the brain size increased relatively suddenly. Scientists credit this change to the discovery of controlled fire. With this discovery, they transitioned from eating raw food to fire-cooked food, which is easier to digest. Thus, eating cooked food allowed them much better nourishment from smaller amounts of food, and their body and brain sizes grew. It is said that primates would not have evolved into humans, at least in our current form, without cooked food. *So, what is the message?* Again, moderation. There are fruits and some vegetables that may be better eaten raw. But, it is much better for your health to eat cooked food as we traditionally do. Certainly, protein quality in these foods increases when eaten in cooked form. A word of caution: cooking is not the same as overcooking, which kills many nutrients such as vitamins.

Now you know that proteins are important in a weight-loss diet. But, I suspect you already eat proteins. How and what could you change? In fact, there is plenty to strategize, and we will see that in the next chapters. But, for starters, let me mention one simple yet very effective trick. I call it *the Protein Shield*. Now, it's your turn to play Doctor. Let me ask you a question based on what you have already read so far. See the following diet followed by Vinita, a non-vegetarian, well-to-do middle-aged homemaker, with two children, who did not enjoy extensive socialization. She was attempting to lose weight even before she came to me. She tried to stick to a diet she had received from a friend, but was miserable with hunger during the day. Her typical food diary before starting my diet plan was as follows:

7 a.m., Breakfast: Tea, 3 idlis or 1 bowl breakfast cereal; 10 a.m.: fruit juice or 2 fruits; 12:30 p.m., Lunch: 1 sandwich with coconut or coriander chutney, a few pieces of dhokla, leftover vegetables from previous night, 2 sticks of carrot; 3:30 p.m.: Tea with 7 Monaco biscuits; 8 p.m.: Some savoury snack such as sev or bhujiya; 9:30 p.m., Dinner with husband: Chicken or fish (a few pieces) or egg bhurjee, daal, roti, curds, little vegetables often with paneer; Bed time: 10:30 p.m.– 6:30 a.m.

Now, please scan the diet and try to spot foods which have a good amount of protein. Remember, eggs, non-vegetarian foods, milk and milk products and daal, are good sources of protein. What do you see? Vinita seems to be eating good sources of proteins. Right? Now, go back to her food diary again and notice the timing. What time is she eating protein foods? Did you notice that most of the good sources of protein are eaten during dinner?

All the wonderful protein foods Vinita was eating were indeed making her full and helping her stay full. But, much of that Protein Shield was operating during her sleep at night. She did not need the Protein Shield during sleep, after all, she was sleeping. So, the protein was going waste at dinner time.

And during the day, when she needed proteins the most, she was hardly eating any. What would you do in this case?

My first order of business was to start her day with a good source of protein such as eggs. I recommended that she save chicken or fish from the previous night for her lunch (instead of only vegetables) and added a bowl of boiled mung/channa in the evening at around 5 p.m. Strategically placing protein-containing foods during daytime truly offered her the Protein Shield from hunger pangs and cravings. The breakfast eggs helped in the morning. The non-vegetarian food at lunch made her mid-day relatively hunger-free and proteins from the bowl of channa or mung in the evening stopped her cravings for high-calorie savoury foods and snacks in the evening, and everyone lived happily – or at least a little thinner – ever after.

So, one more time:

- Proteins are hugely important for our body, our survival and well-being.
- The Indian diet is generally low in protein, and Indians have lower muscle mass compared to people from Western countries.
- Eating foods containing proteins is the only way to give your body proteins.
- Eggs, non-vegetarian foods, milk, daals, beans, pulses are good sources of protein.
- Protein Power can be harnessed especially for weight loss.

- Eating good amount of protein (not too high)
  —helps you feel full
  —increases the proportion of fat loss
  —reduces the risk of weight regain

- The Protein Shield can be used strategically by timing protein intake to minimize hunger and cravings during the day.

3

Preparing for the Diet

Losing weight and keeping it off is not an easy journey. The road bends, dips, rises and crosses many paths. It's not easy and there are no guarantees. However, I know the road, I know the dangerous turns as well as resting places on this road. I have crossed it with my patients thousands of times. Through this book, I will hold your hand and we will make that journey. I will walk you through one step at a time. Your job is to follow the steps. The next chapter deals with the actual diet that you could use for weight loss but before embarking on that diet, you need to follow these three steps.

Step 1: Get ready
Step 2: Let the doctor in
Step 3: Line up the tools

Let me elaborate a bit.

Step 1: Get ready

The first important 'action item' for you is to decide if this is the *right time* for you to start a weight loss programme.

Are you really ready, or just excited in the moment? If you're not ready, it's better not to try. The reality is, despite all the promises you may have read in other diet books or read on the internet, losing a substantial amount of weight and keeping it off is not easy.

To lose weight, or more specifically to lose stored fat from the body, you have to eat less food than your body needs. And, you have to continue to eat less for weeks, possibly months. It will need dedication and commitment. Is *now* the time you are ready take on this commitment? Are you willing to make long term changes to your diet and lifestyle?

Once I had a patient from a royal family. His weight was nearing 110 kg. I asked him the question, 'Are you ready to lose weight?'

'Of course,' he replied, 'I have three cooks who can cook anything you write for me. You write and I follow.'

Wow. This is what I call commitment, I thought. Then he mentioned his only condition. He drank an entire bottle of scotch and twenty-two bottles of Coca Cola (there was no Diet Coke those days) every day. He did not want to reduce his scotch or Coke, but was prepared to reduce food a bit. Clearly, this was not going to work. A reasonable amount of alcohol could certainly be accommodated in a weight-loss diet. But, not a full bottle of scotch, every single day, let alone those bottles of sugary-sweet water. He was not ready, even though he said so. I told him to come back if and when he was mentally prepared to embark on a diet and make some more compromises. What do you think would have happened had he started the diet programme? You already know the answer. He would not have lost much weight. But, that is not the worst part. In this case, the diet would receive the blame and he would have been convinced that 'diets don't work for him'. Typically, people write off forever the weight-loss approach that they were trying. Therefore, it is much better to not start the programme if you are not in the right mindset.

Recently, a patient asked me about helping his son who was in his early twenties, living in Singapore, away from parents. The son struggled with weight and had been diagnosed with diabetes. The father was very concerned about his son's health and knew very well that weight loss would immensely help his diabetes. My response was to first check with his son if he was ready to undertake a diet programme. The son responded that he was willing to diet on Mondays, Tuesdays and the first half of Wednesdays. Other days of the week were filled with social commitments and parties. Needless to say, he was not ready.

How do you know when you are ready?

Sometimes, you may have the right mindset, but not the right situation in life – a very busy time at work, illness of a relative you are caring for, approaching exams or travel are some of the reasons that people tend to put off their diet programme. Here, I would like to draw a distinction. The right *mindset* and the right *situation* are two separate things.

You should not embark on a weight loss programme without the right mindset. However, that is not the same with the right situation. If you wait for the 'right time' in your life, it is hard to come by. For example, we have year round festivals in India which serve as reasons to avoid starting a diet. First, it would be the wedding season, Christmas, the New Year, Holi, kids' exams, summer vacations, monsoons, the October heat, Navratri, Diwali and on and on. If you don't break the cycle somewhere and take the plunge, there will never be a suitable time to diet.

There is one more reason for initiating a programme sooner rather than later. Whether in a photo album or on Facebook, think of how you feel when you see a photo of yourself from the past. You wonder how different you used to look. So young! Your perception is accurate. The reality is, we are all ageing daily. Every day, you look older than the day before, but younger than what you will look five or ten years from today. So, today is the day to look your youngest. Just the same, when it comes to weight loss, today is your day. With age, our ability to lose weight decreases and it becomes easier and easier to gain weight. Even though you may have struggled with weight all your life, when you were twenty-five, you could perhaps cut down a bit on your diet, here and there, and lose 4 or 5 kg easily. Not so when you are thirty-five, forty-five or fifty-five years old. You will have to put in *much* more effort than you did as a young twenty-something. But, look at this as glass half full. If *this* is the effort needed at forty-five, imagine what it would take to lose weight at fifty-five? Or, if you are at fifty-five, what would you do at sixty-five? Whatever your current age, compared to the future you, age is on your side *right now*.

You have the right mindset, but the situation around you is not right?

You can modify the situation to the best of your ability. In my experience, at times, the greatest danger to adhering to a diet plan is not you, but your well-meaning friends and relatives. When you attend your friend's daughter's birthday party, do you hear the admonitions to, 'Keep your diet at home,' or, 'You are not going to diet today, enjoy the birthday and start tomorrow.' Or my favourite, 'What? Such little food? No seconds? You didn't like our food?' Surely, you have heard some version of these. It is not easy to control the temptation to eat. And when faced with this kind of social onslaught, most of us tend to drop our resistance and give in to temptation. In a subsequent chapter, we will see how to deal with such social landmines. However, to get you started on a diet plan, the best approach is to anticipate these landmines and confront them.

Start with your family. Talk with your husband or wife, parents, siblings, children, maybe even other relatives in your home. Let them know that what you are about to start is very important for your health and that you need their support and help in achieving it. Let them know that it is a challenging task as it is. You would appreciate if certain food that is not right for you does not enter the house, if possible. In general, your family does not need to be punished because of your diet. If the sweets do come in, ask that they don't leave the boxes of chocolates or mithai lying on the dining table. For you, this will be out of sight and out of mind. All you are asking of your family is sensitivity around the fact that you will be on a diet that may not include all the high-calorie foods that they may eat.

Next in line are your friends and relatives. For example, if you have some close friends whom you meet often, start by recruiting their help in your efforts to lose weight. Let them know your 'weak points' when it comes to food. Mention how they could specifically help. You may recruit their help to not tempt you with food or taunt about your diet, or even join you for walking or other activity. Yes, that also means that you will have to be upfront about your efforts to lose weight and improve your health. There is no hiding it. Imagine someone with diabetes who needs insulin injections trying to hide the treatment? It's not necessary, and you won't be able to successfully hide it. Same goes for this situation. Even if there's a chance you may not totally succeed, it is better to be open about it. A bit about human nature: if someone asks for help, we are wired to respond positively. You do need the help of your family, relatives and friends in accomplishing your diet goal. So, confide in them to make them participants in your programme, making them small stakeholders in your success. This team approach works quite well.

The last on the list for preparing your mind for the diet is to discard all weight-loss secrets that you may have previously heard. I bet you have heard at least one of the following as the best treatment for weight loss: honey and lime, lime and warm water, ghee, egg white instead of whole egg, roti instead of rice, warm food instead of cold, karela (bitter gourd), home-grown instead of organic, avoiding root vegetables, and many more. There is no scientific evidence to support these. If you continue to harbour these notions, you may not be able to follow the diet programme suggested in the next chapter. So, wipe your slate clean, and start this programme.

Now that you've decided you're ready to start. Let's move on to Step 2.

Step 2: Let the doctor in

Some years back, when I was in Goa, I met Mrs Sunita. She was thirty-two years old and wanted to lose weight before having children. Her first claim was that she was completely healthy except for the weight. But her somewhat puffy face, thinning hair and eyebrows, slightly hoarse voice were telling the doctor in me something. I asked her do you feel colder than others? Do you have dry skin? Constipation? As expected, she said yes. She was surprised that I 'guessed' these things about her. But it wasn't a guess. I let her know that all these symptoms, including some weight gain, were signs of her thyroid hormone not functioning adequately. Sure enough, a blood test indicated that she had a very poorly functioning thyroid. Fortunately, medication could correct that easily. I am glad that we discovered her thyroid issue. Low thyroid function (unless corrected by medication) can slow down your weight loss. However, more seriously for Sunita, who wished to become pregnant, not correcting her thyroid deficiency could have had adverse effects on the baby.

Now, only some people have low thyroid levels, and not everyone with excess weight suffers from it. But this case highlights an important point. Improving health through weight loss requires a nutritional approach *as well as* medical support. For another example, consider the link between weight loss and sleep. Inadequate or poor quality sleep contributes to weight gain. When poor sleep may be a culprit in weight, you need to see a physician specializing in sleep disorders. If the sleep disorder remains untreated, the weight-loss effort may not be very successful. Yet another reason to involve your physician is to monitor your health improvement as you lose weight. Those who have diabetes or high blood sugar or high blood pressure may be on medications. Scientific weight loss would almost certainly improve these conditions. As your blood sugar improves or blood pressure drops, it may become necessary to reduce the dose of those medications.

Your physician can help you monitor the conditions and set the new dose.

Ideally, you need someone who knows medicine to take care of your health and gives guidance about diet and nutrition. Unfortunately, medical colleges do not teach much about nutrition and, typically, dietitians or nutritionists are not doctors. Thus, it is extremely rare to find such a combination. Fortunately, I have received formal training as a doctor as well as in nutrition. However, I am not treating you as a doctor. Consider me as your nutritionist, helping you through this book. Now, it would be nice if you pair this book up with your physician. Feel free to share this book with your doctor. Let him or her know that you are starting this scientific weight-loss programme. I hope this emphasizes the medical aspect of improving your health through the management of your weight and related medical conditions. Although you may not have seen such a recommendation in diet books, just like you recruited your family and friends, recruit your physician into this team effort.

Thus, Step 2 for you to start this diet programme is to let your doctor know about it.

Step 3: Time to prepare

Find out how much excess weight you have: This is a last bit of homework before starting the diet. A top question on your mind may be 'how much weight should I lose?' This is in fact two questions rolled into one. The first question is how overweight am I? The second question is: how much should you lose? Body mass index, or BMI, is the most common and reliable way to answer both questions. BMI is an indirect measurement of the fat in your body – higher the BMI, greater the fat.

You could either use the BMI calculator at www.dhurandhar.com. Or, calculate as follows:

1. Measure your weight in kg and height in cm. Let's say your weight is 75 kg. If your height is 157 cm, or 1.57 metres.
2. To calculate BMI, divide your weight (75 kg) by your height (1.57)
3. Take the answer, and divide by your height (1.57) again. The answer is 30.4, which is your BMI.

The formula to calculate BMI is the same for adults of all ages. It also does not depend on your bone structure, whether you are broad-boned or otherwise. For Asians and people from the Indian subcontinent, a *BMI ranging 18 to 23 is considered 'normal', from 23-25 is considered as overweight and above 25 is considered as obesity.* As your weight drops, the BMI will decrease. As from the above example, if weight drops to 70 kg, that weight divided by 1.57 and again by 1.57 will give you the BMI of 28.39. In other words, at that height of 1.57

metres, your will need to reach about 60kg to achieve a BMI below 25.

Determine how much weight to lose: This is the second question. Ideally, for Indians / Asians, one could aim to reach to BMI around 23. However, it may neither be possible, nor necessary. Each one of us responds differently to a diet. It is hard to predict how much weight you will lose and how fast. So, it may not be completely under your control to reach the BMI of 23 or any other BMI that you may desire. Those of us who have the 'tendency' to gain weight may never become rail thin. But again, it is not even necessary. Instead of asking how much weight I should lose, a better question is to ask is 'What would be a reasonable goal to aim for?' Research has indicated that if you lose just 5 to 10 per cent of body weight, you will considerably improve health even if you don't look like a supermodel. *If your starting weight is 80 kg, losing just 4 to 8 kg may improve diabetes or blood pressure, cholesterol or backache.* Therefore, my recommendation is to consider weight loss a stepwise process. In step 1, your goal should be to lose 5 per cent weight, i.e., 4 kg if you are 80 kg, 5 kg if you are 100 kg to start with, and so on. After you reach your first goal, if you need further weight loss and are up to it, step 2 would be to lose the next 5 per cent. This approach also makes the task manageable and not overwhelming.

Remember, maintaining that lost weight is equally important, which we will review in a subsequent chapter. *But, for now, let's aim for a 5 per cent weight loss.*

Determine how many calorie diet you will need to lose weight. The next chapter gives sample diets of various calorie levels. But which one is good for you? Here's how you decide that. First, let's calculate the approximate number of calories you require in a day. We will do this in two steps.

First calculate your basal metabolic requirement (BMR) of calories. Simply stated, BMR is the minimum number of calories needed in a day to stay alive, if you decide to just lie in bed and sleep the whole day. Second, consider your physical activity and add the appropriate number of calories to BMR to arrive at the calories needed for the day. So, let's get started. You will need a calculator for this step, or you can use the free calculator at www.dhurandhar.com.

Calculate your BMR

For women:

655 + (9.57 x weight in kg) + (4.7 x height in inches) - (4.7 x age in years)

BMR =

For Men:

66 + (13.7 x weight in kg) + (12.7 x height in inches) - (6.8 x age in years)

BMR =

2. Total calorie requirement based on your activity

Multiply your BMR (from step 1 above) by the activity factor, as follows:

Table 1: Computing Calorie requirement

If your activity is	Multiply BMR by this number
Sedentary (desk job, minimal walking, very light work in the house)	1.2 *
Light activity (light activity such as 30 to 50 min walking or similar activity a day, for 1 to 3 times a week)	1.375 *
Moderate activity (cardio training, dancing, jogging, swimming 30 min to 60 min per day, 3 to 5 times a week)	1.55
Very active (very high level of activity almost every day of the week, such as 60 min biking or high activity sports such as badminton, football, basketball)	1.725

If your activity is	Multiply BMR by this number
Super active

(very hard exercise or training such as training for a marathon, competitive swimming, long hikes several times a week) | 1.9 |
| * Although it is very tempting to consider yourself as an active person, most of us are likely to be either sedentary or with light activity. | |

Now, let's take an example and calculate the total calorie need for Nina, a forty-year-old computer programmer with limited need to do physical work in the house or at office, whose weight is 75 kg and height is 5 feet and 3 inches (63 inches). Let's plug these numbers in the formula for women.

655 + [9.57 x 75 (weight)] = 655 + 717.75 = 1372.75

+ [4.7 x 63 (height)] = 296.1

- [4.7 x 40 (age)] = 188

BMR = 1372.75 + 296.1 − 188 = 1480.85

Step 2: Multiply the BMR with 1.2 (sedentary activity) = 1480 x 1.2 = 1776 calories.

As a sedentary person,. Nina needs 1776 calories per day. Instead, if she were a person with light activity, she would multiply her BMR with 1.375, instead of 1.2. So, her daily need of calories would be 1480 x 1.375 = 2035.

If all this math is too much for you, there are many websites that can calculate your daily requirement for you. You simply need to enter your gender (male / female), age, height and weight. Here is a website for your convenience: www.Dhurandhar.com

As a quick fun activity, let's consider two other scenarios for Nina. In the previous parameters, she needs 1,776 calories a day. The above formula can tell us her calorie requirement if she were sixty years of age. Even if her weight remains the same, Nina's BMR would be 1386 and total calorie need would be 1664 calories, when she is sixty. That is less by about 110 calories per day, or about 3300 calories per month. You can now see how our calorie need drops with age, which makes it easier to gain weight as our age advances. Therefore, in many ways, the best day in your life to start the diet is today.

Another scenario is her calorie need after weight loss. What happens if Nina loses 10 kg? At 65 kg and at the same age, she will start requiring about 100 fewer calories per day. This also means that to keep losing weight, one has to keep reducing calorie intake as the weight drops. This is one reason why your weight loss slows down after a while if your diet is not reduced appropriately.

Now that you know your calorie need for the day, it is easy to determine the diet you will use for weight loss. It should be about 400 to 500 calories less than your requirement for the day. So, if your total daily calorie need is 2600 calories, start a weight loss diet of about 2200 calories. If your need is 1800, start a diet with 1400 calories. I would rarely recommend to start on a diet less than 1400 calories. So, if your calorie need turns out to be say 1600 calories per day, start with a 1400 calorie diet (and not 1200 calories).

Table 2: Selecting calories for your weight-loss diet

If your calorie need for the day is	Select the weight loss diet of
1700 or less	1400 calories
1800 – 2100	1700 calories
2200 – 2400	1900 calories
2500 – 3000	2200 calories

Gather your tools: You are going to need certain tools during your journey to lose weight. The most basic requirement is a weighing scale, or what is popularly known as the bathroom scale. It is important that your weighing scale is in good working order. If it is very old, it can shows erratic readings. It would be best to invest in a new, decent scale. If you can afford, an even better investment would be a scale that measures your body fat. This is also known as a bio-electrical impedance scale or a BIA scale. It can be ordered over the internet and costs a little more than Rs 3,000. It looks like a bathroom scale and just like the weighing scale, you stand on it. It gives your reading for weight and fat percentage. As we have previously discussed, it is important to focus on fat loss instead of weight loss. Obviously, you will need to know fat percentage, if you wish to track changes in fat.

Another scale that you will also find useful is a kitchen scale. Something that weighs 20, 50, 100 or 200 g. This is to weigh your food. As you will see in the next chapter, it is inaccurate to write a diet that specifies the number, such as two chapattis or four rotis, etc. The number of chapatis could be misleading, as the size and thickness of the rotis may vary with household. Therefore, it is best to specify the weight of wheat flour (aata) in a diet. Use the kitchen scale to weigh that flour on day 1, and note the number of rotis you make. Once you note this, you will not have to weigh flour every day.

Another useful gadget for your programme is a pedometer. This is an instrument that counts the number of steps you walk. It comes in many shapes and sizes. Earlier versions included a small box, the size of a matchbox, which you could tuck in your pant/sari at your waist. Nowadays, most smartphones have apps that will measure your steps. Perhaps, the most useful are Fitbit, Vivofit or similar pedometers, which are like a wristwatch. In fact, they also show the time, in addition to showing the steps or the distance you walked in a day. I use a Vivofit and my goal is to complete at least 10,000 steps every single day. It is Sunday night, and I have been writing for a long time. While writing this, I happened to glance at my Vivofit. It shows 8,445 steps so far. Not quite

10,000. However, the wind outside is howling, as it often is in West Texas where we live, and the temperature is hovering around 3° Celsius. So, I will push myself to walk in our house to complete the remaining 1,555 steps before going to bed. The number stares in your face. There is no guesswork and no escaping the fact that the quota for the day is not complete. I think this motivation to achieve your daily target is a great benefit of using a pedometer to monitor your steps for the day. You should have one too.

The final 'tool' you will need is a good measuring tape that is non-stretchable. Try pulling it and it should not stretch. This is for recording your body measurements, so your progress can be tracked. Sometimes, due to water retention, your weighing scale may mask your actual fat loss. At such times, body measurements are excellent in indicating progress. For example, if in two weeks, your weighing scale shows a loss of only 200 g, but a reduction of 1" from the waist and ½" from the hips, you should realize that there has been substantial fat loss. The tape measures need to be taken at the same spot, preferably directly over the skin (and not clothes), same time of the day and by you, not someone else. This is because the measurement can vary if you change the location or squeeze the tape too tight or loose.

Track your progress: As a final step of the preparation, get ready to track your progress as presented in this table.

Table 3: Weekly weight-loss chart

Week	Weight (kg)	Fat per cent	Waist (inches)	Hips (inches)	Thigh (inches)	Chest (inches)	Arm (inches)	Neck (inches)
Start								
2								
4								
6								
8								
10								
12								

Here are some helpful hints related to each of these markers of progress:

Table 4: Some helpful hints

How often	Note these markers once in two weeks. The measurements fluctuate, hence can be misleading if noted more frequently.
Weighing scale	Weigh at same time of the day. Morning is preferable. Use same clothes or same level of undressing. Weighing scale placed on a carpet or uneven surface could give inaccurate reading. Old machines or dying batteries could give misleading numbers.
BIA machine for fat per cent	Measure same time of the day, preferably in the morning, after passing urine. Make sure the machine is set to right gender (male / female) – else, this can give huge error.
Waist measurement	Stand erect, preferably no clothing on measurement area. Place the tape around waist at the level of belly button (umbilicus) and wrap around firmly but not too tight to squeeze the skin. Note that some fluctuations can occur on the days when stomach is bloated due to gas.
Hip measurement	Stand erect, preferably no clothing on measurement area. Place the tape around hips where it gives maximum reading. Wrap around firmly but not too tight to squeeze the skin.

Thigh measurement	Sit on the edge of a chair. Expose the area of measurement. Measure 5" towards the waist from the top of the knee cap. At that point, measure the circumference of the thigh.
Chest measurement	Stand erect. Pass the tape around your chest at the level of nipples. Breath out. Measure without taking a breath and while pressing firmly, but without pinching the skin.
Arm measurement	Sit or stand. If right handed, fold left hand. Measure 4" towards the shoulder from your left elbow. At that point, measure the circumference of the arm.
Neck measurement	Stand without looking down or up. Look straight ahead, pass the tape around your neck and measure while pressing firmly but without pinching skin at the base of your neck (where neck joins the shoulder).

Summary and Checklist

Losing fat is a serious undertaking. In some situations, it is a battle. Don't engage the enemy if you are not ready. Take on the enemy at a time of your choosing and on your terms, but don't delay. To go to this battle well prepared, form alliances, be well informed, well determined and well equipped. Here is a checklist to help you get ready:

1. Get ready—
   Ask the following questions to yourself:

a. Are you ready to take on this commitment now?
b. Are you willing to make long-term changes to your diet and lifestyle?

If the answer is Yes, then take the following steps:

c. Ask your family to help improve your health.
d. Openly and candidly recruit the help of your friends.
e. Clear your mind of all the wrong notions that you have heard or read about weight loss.

1. Let your doctor know about the programme you are about to start.
2. Get your numbers.
    a. The excess weight you have: _____
    b. How much weight you should lose: _____
    c. The calories needed for your weight-loss diet: _____
4. Get the tools:
    a. weighing scale,
    b. BIA scale for body fat measurement,
    c. kitchen scale,
    d. pedometer, and
    e. measuring tape.
5. Chart to record your progress.

Your diet starts in the next chapter. Best of luck!

4

Protein Power Diet Plan

You might have heard or read that by 'just eating healthy' you can get rid of obesity. Forget it! You will not. There is *no* scientific evidence to support this 'feel good' statement. The next time you hear someone claim that, ask for the evidence. They won't have any. There is none. If you wish to lose fat, you must eat fewer calories than you need. No diet, no fat loss. Exercise without diet will not produce fat loss for most of us. This chapter will offer you low calorie diet plans that are reasonable, practical, flexible and sustainable. I have personally worked with thousands of individuals who have successfully followed similar diet plans tailor-made to their requirements.

There are three objectives in developing these 'Protein-Power' low-calorie diet plans that I am sharing with you below. 1) Adequacy: These diet plans are low in calories, yet they provide key nutrients needed for health. 2) Applicability: While it is difficult to personalize a diet plan in a book to match every individual personality possible, these diets are built in such a way that they apply to a large number of people. 3) Quality of life: Dieting for fat loss does take serious commitment and efforts. However, a well-selected diet should not leave you hungry and miserable the whole day. It should neither be boring nor a punishment. Quite the contrary. Foods in these diet plans are strategically placed so you will feel full and hunger will not drive you crazy. Various food options suggested give you choice and variation.

Ten Components of a Healthful Diet for Weight Loss

So, let's get started. First, let me describe to you the key components of these diets.

1. **Water:** Water is life! It's even more important to drink plenty of water when on a weight-loss diet. It helps carry nutrients as well as waste products of metabolism, helps soften stools and prevents constipation – which is a frequent complaint experienced because food quantity is reduced. Drinking water also replaces water lost as sweat when you start an exercise programme. Most importantly, water has an almost magical property of fullness, only if timed correctly. Here is an experiment you can try today: Drink a full glass of water and five minutes later eat a snack or your breakfast. Note the feeling of fullness on a scale of 1 to 10. One being not full at all and 10 being the most full you have ever felt. Now, tomorrow, eat the exact same breakfast at the same time. But, this time, drink the same amount of water in the middle of the breakfast or right after. Note the feeling

of fullness. I bet you feel way fuller when you drink water during or after a meal than drinking the same amount before a meal. This fact has actually been supported by research. Let's use this principle to our advantage. As you approach the end of your meal, drink a full glass of water. You will instantly feel full and all other thoughts about eating additional food will disappear. You may have heard that one should not drink water with a meal. The conventional wisdom behind that adage is that you will eat less food if you drink water. In our case, that is the point!

2. **Cell-healthy fats**: Fat, oil, ghee, butter and cream are equivalent to 'bad words' in a dieter's dictionary. Collectively, these are called 'fat' in nutrition. Fact is that fat is an essential component of our body, skin, brain, cells and cell cover known as the cell membrane. Therefore, eating a certain amount of fat is necessary. It is also true that fat has more than double the number of calories compared to carbohydrates or proteins. A roasted papad has about 30 calories. When fried, calories in that same papad can be about 150, all thanks to the oil in which it was fried. In a weight-loss diet, you need to be really mindful of the amount of oil used for cooking. In this sense, your success is at the mercy of the person who cooks in your household. If you have a cook, it is extremely important that this person prepares food in the given amount of oil quota for you. Oil is such an invisible

nutrient that you will be unable to tell the amount of oil used once the food is cooked.

A real story: one of my patients had two households, in the Middle East and in Mumbai, and he alternated stays for several weeks at a time in a place for business. After a while I noticed a pattern. This patient lost weight well when in the Middle East but not at all when in Mumbai. After thinking it through, I brought up the possibility of oil usage to the attention of this patient. At first he was confident that there was no mistake in oil usage as he had instructed the cooks in both cities to be careful about it. Turns out, when confronted, the cook in Mumbai admitted to using oil liberally. Funnily enough, the cook refused to use less oil. In the cook's opinion, food did not taste good with less oil. In many ways, his job depended on using oil to make tasty food to please his boss. The cook did end up losing his job. This is only one of the ways I get to play a diet-and-lifestyle detective in my role as a nutritionist. I listen, watch, read very carefully when interacting with patients. I read between the lines and hear the unsaid. It pays off.

3. **Bone-friendly milk**: Forget the rumour that milk is not good for adults. It is true that a few people are unable to digest milk sugar, known as lactose. They get an upset stomach or gas with milk. This is described as lactose intolerance. If you are not one of those – most people have

no difficulty in digesting milk – milk has good quality protein and calcium, which is important for the bone health of Indians, who have a widespread tendency to have brittle bones. If you eat curds, it is even better. You will get all the benefits of milk in terms of calcium and protein. In addition, curds will have gut-friendly bacteria which are helpful for your intestines and general health.

4. **Start-right breakfast**: Skipping breakfast does not enable faster weight loss. You tend to build hunger and will end up eating the same amount or more, by the end of the day. Instead, it is better to start your day with breaking your overnight fast, but with only a limited portion size.

5. **Protein shield**: We've already discussed in the previous chapter how eating protein increases fullness and protects you from feeling hungry. Strategically placed protein snacks at mid-morning and late afternoon protect you from excessive hunger and cravings during the day and at night, respectively.

6. **Brain energy**: I am referring to foods that are a good source of carbohydrates. Our brain almost exclusively depends on carbohydrates for energy. We need carbohydrates. The staples in an Indian diet – roti, chapati, rice, naan, paratha, etc. – are good and important sources of carbohydrates. Some people have turned carbohydrates into a dirty word. A line of thinking has emerged that condemns good sources of carbohydrates such as wheat. Interestingly, this resentment is actually targeted towards gluten, a protein

(not carbohydrate) in cereals like wheat, rye or barley. It is true that some people (less than 1 in 100), respond adversely to gluten and get bad stomach and intestinal symptoms. These individuals feel better by eating gluten-free foods. However, gluten can be handled easily and very well by the remaining 99 of 100 individuals. Asking everyone to quit eating sources of carbohydrates such as wheat is like asking everyone to stop eating peanuts or strawberries because some individuals are allergic to these foods. Those who are not allergic to strawberry will not benefit from avoiding strawberries.

While on this topic, it is worth differentiating between complex carbohydrates such as those that you get from wheat, rice, cereals and vegetables from simple carbohydrates such as table sugar or foods high in sugar such as soft drinks. Besides calories, sugar does not provide any other nutrient. Also, unlike the sugar from complex carbohydrates, these sugars cause an immediate spike in blood sugar levels. Hence, even though carbohydrates are important for us, there is no particular reason for eating high sugar foods beyond moderation.

Soluble fibres: Technically, fibres are a part of carbohydrates. The two types of fibres in diet are soluble and insoluble. Insoluble fibres comes from wheat bran, seeds and skins of fruits. Important source of soluble fibre are vegetables, mainly, the green leafy vegetables. You must have heard about the importance of fibre in preventing constipation, and in reducing the risk of cancer or heart disease. The credit for this mainly goes to soluble fibre. Indians can also use vegetables as a source of iron.

7. **Muscle-saver protein**: The previous chapter discussed how proteins in diet can help protect you from muscle loss. In addition, the use of protein foods in lunch or dinner greatly helps in remaining full for a longer time.

8. **Fruity vitamins**: Fruits provide fibre and vitamins. As such, vegetables also have some vitamins. However, the process of rinsing and cooking vegetables can destroy a large amount of those vitamins. Fruits on the other hand are eaten raw, right after cutting them. Do not expose cut fruits to air and light for a long time as it can reduce their vitamin content.

9. **Fun stuff:** This one is to make your diet interesting. A small treat for yourself, at the end of a diet day, especially for those with a sweet tooth. But there is another reason. There seems to be some useful purpose in the tradition of ending a meal with a dessert. We tested the concept in animal research and discovered that eating something sweet increases fullness. Thus, eating a small amount of sweet at the end of the dinner will top off your fullness, and you will be ready to stop eating for the day.

I successfully use this concept for those who have lost weight and are maintaining it. I recommend that before going to a wedding, or a party, where you are anticipating a heavy meal, drink a cup of tea or coffee with sugar. The sweet beverage substantially curbs your desire to indulge.

A couple of points to note: Do not overdo the 'fun stuff' part. Remember moderation. Most desserts are indeed calorie dense, that is, they pack in more calories per gram. And, most of these calories in desserts come from their fat content, not sugar. It is the fat in them that is giving the bad name for sweet tasting desserts, not sugar. It is quite fashionable to malign sugar. People have tried selling books by claiming sugar is our enemy. However, a careful review of scientific literature fails to show what damage sugar does in the area of body weight regulation that is beyond its calorie value. Even the oft-cited report on the amount of sugar in diet from the World Health Organization admits that in many ways there is limited evidence to blame sugar. Sugar is a simple carbohydrate and should not be consumed in excess as noted above. However, calorie-wise, it is less harmful than fats in the food. Fat has more than twice the calories of sugar. Hence, worry about how much oil / ghee or cream is in jalebi, ras malai, cake or ice cream rather than just plain sugar.

Another point worth mentioning here is about artificial sweeteners or sugar substitutes. There is no scientific basis to consider currently available sweeteners such as Splenda or Equal harmful. Yet, that has not stopped some proponents to give the sugar substitutes a bad name. As in other quackery, a proponent latches on to a grain of truth and spins theories that have no scientific basis. For example, it is claimed that aspartame, which is sold as Equal or Nutrasweet, is dangerous. In fact, aspartame is simply a combination of two amino acids (components of protein), aspartic acid and phenylalanine. Of these, phenylalanine is avoided if someone has a rare condition called phenylketonurea (PKU). It has no adverse effect if you don't have PKU (and almost none of you will have it). Furthermore, it is claimed that aspartame is converted to methanol and then to formic acid. Sounds terrible, right? What is usually left out to mention is that methanol is also a part of our normal regular diet, including fruits and vegetables.

So, the case in point: If you wish to use a sugar substitute, go ahead. You will save calories from sugar. I like my fruits sweet. I carry chopped fruits for lunch that are mixed with Splenda. Sweet taste, minus the calories.

The Diet

Now, with this preparation, here are the next steps. As outlined in the previous chapter, determine the calorie value of a diet that you would like to follow. Say, it is 1700 calories. Now, look at Tables 5 for the diet prescription for 1700 calories. The first three rows address the amounts you can have for the entire day. Tea or coffee, milk and the cooking oil quota for the entire day. This is followed by the meals throughout the day, starting with breakfast at say 7 a.m., followed by a mid-morning snack at 10 or 10.30 a.m. and lunch around noon or 1 p.m. Note that your mid-morning meal (such as nuts) is to provide a daytime protein shield. Also, notice the different important components of a healthful lunch. For many Indians, the gap between lunch and dinner is too long, and that is also a danger zone for dieting. You could have your usual tea/coffee at say 3 or 4 p.m., but what you really need at this time is the second protection of protein shield, say in the form of a protein shake. You will end the day with a wholesome dinner and a small, fun stuff treat for yourself. Finally, remember to drink a glass of water immediately after lunch and dinner, or towards the end of a meal.

Table 5: The diet chart

Food and meals	1400 Calories	1700 Calories	1900 Calories	2200 Calories
Tea/coffee	Without sugar; Use sugar substitutes such as Splenda, Stevia, Sweet 'n Low			
Bone-friendly skimmed milk	1.5 cup	2 cups	2 cups	2.5 cups
Cell-healthy fat	3 teaspoons	4 teaspoons	4 teaspoons	5 teaspoons
Start right breakfast	Whole egg 1 (any preparation) 2 bread slices 2 teaspoons jam Or, select from the choices in Table xxx			
Protein shield mid-day	Nuts 30 g	Nuts 30 g	Nuts 30 g	Nuts 30 g

Lunch	1 glass of water immediately after lunch			
Brain energy	1 Roti	1 Roti	2 Rotis	3 Rotis
Muscle-saver protein	Pulses 25 g	Pulses 50 g	Pulses 50 g	Pulses 50 g
Soluble fibre	Vegetables 200 g	Vegetables 200 g	Vegetables 200 g	Vegetables 200 g
Fruity vitamins units	1 Fruit	1 Fruit	1 Fruit	2 Fruits
Protein shield - night	½ scoop protein shake	½ scoop protein shake	1 scoop protein shake	1 scoop protein shake
Dinner	1 glass of water immediately after dinner			
Brain energy	1 Roti	2 Rotis	3 Rotis	3 Rotis
Muscle-saver protein	Pulses 25 g	Pulses 50 g	Pulses 50 g	Pulses 50 g
Soluble fibre	Vegetables 200 g	Vegetables 200 g	Vegetables 200 g	Vegetables 200 g
Fruity vitamins	1 Fruit	1 Fruit	1 Fruit	1 Fruit
Fun stuff	1 small scoop ice cream			

What are some options and substitutions?

What if you want some change, some different options or replacements? Yes, you can certainly consider some options as outlined in Table 6.

Let's review these options individually. For every one cup of skimmed milk from your diet, you could replace with equal amount of soy milk, curds, etc. Of the two cups of milk recommended for a 1700 calorie diet, you could use one cup milk for preparing tea/coffee and the remaining one cup could be replaced with soy milk, curds, or even ice cream made with one cup milk, some sweetener such as Splenda or Stevia and some fruits such as strawberries added for fun and taste.

Table 6 shows some options for breakfast. You could replace the breakfast with either one of the foods listed. For example, one day you could have the egg and bread breakfast, next day roti and vegetables and the day after upma or poha. A VERY IMPORTANT point: The size, style and thickness of chapatis/rotis/parathas will vary with each household. Therefore, the number of rotis without mentioning the weight of flour could be misleading. The roti mentioned here is from 25 g of wheat flour (aata). You will have to weigh 25 or 50 g aata on day 1 and determine the number of rotis, phulka or naan or chapatis that your household makes. Once you know the number, you need not weigh flour daily. The same holds true for poha, upma, rice or other foods where the weight is mentioned. The weight is of the food in raw condition (raw rice, raw rice flakes – poha).

The mid-day protein shield will provide you a protein-packed small meal of few calories between breakfast and lunch. The options are listed considering convenience. Whether at home or at office, you will not have to cook this meal. You could even stash your work desk or refrigerator with these options of nuts, Greek yogurt, protein bar. This meal will have a strong effect on reducing your hunger at lunch.

Table 6 also provides explanations or substitutions for roti, rice, pulses, vegetables and fruits. Just like the rotis, weigh raw rice first and cook. Once you know the measure (cup, bowl or a katori), you need not weigh rice daily. Consider pulses as an important source of proteins, especially for the vegetarians. These include pulses/beans/lentils such as channa (including roasted channa), rajma, moong, chole, black eyed peas, peas, or other members of this family. You could substitute pulses for non-vegetarian food such as chicken/fish/mutton. Once again, the weights noted for the non-vegetarian food are also raw and without bones. Weigh them once before cooking, so you will get an idea. The last part of Table 6 is about some fun stuff you can have in moderation. Be aware that it would interfere with weight loss if you start taking too much liberty with these foods.

Also, note that all these substitutions are approximations and not an exact equivalent for all nutrients. They are close substitutions for calories. Instead of being super strict and unrealistic about finding an exact match for each nutrient, the effort here is to focus on convenience, and your long-term compliance for best results.

Let's also discuss another crucial aspect – an occasional lapse in diet. If you have been following the diet well, but attended a wedding or a party and ended up eating way more than you should have, what do you do? First, do not despair or be hard on yourself. Try not to go too astray. However, if you do, just try to compensate for the extra calories the next day. Note, I said, 'next day'. I did not say 'that day' or 'the next few days'. This is because most dietary indiscretions happen during dinner. At that time, you do not have diet quota remaining for the day to compensate from. Therefore, try to go somewhat easy on food the next day. However, do not extend this corrective action for several days, as you will then miss out on necessary nutrients for multiple days in a row. The best is not to have cheat days at all, the next best is to limit your cheat days. If indeed you do, then try to compensate only gradually and lightly the next day.

Table 6: Replacements/options

Replacement for 1 cup skimmed milk
1 cup Soy milk
1 cup curds / yogurt
Buttermilk made from 1 cup curd
Ice cream made from 1 cup milk and sugar substitutes
1 cup lactose-free milk
Cream cheese 50 g (2 slices of cheese such as Amul.

Options for breakfast
2 Roti + 200 g vegetables or 100 g potatoes
2 Roti + 25 g chole /sprouts / beans
Upma made from 75 g rawa
Poha made from 75 g rice flakes
4 Idlis (about 3" diameter)
2 Dosa (plain)
Breakfast cereal 1 bowl (e.g. corn flakes) plus 1.5 cup milk

Options for Protein Shield mid-day (30 g Nuts)
15 cashew nuts or 35 ground nuts, 18 almonds
1 slice bread and 1 table spoon peanut butter
1 slice bread and 2 egg whites (the white part of eggs)
Protein bar that provides about 8 to 10 g protein
Greek yogurt
Tomato omelet made from 40 g besan and ½ teaspoon oil

Substitution for 1 roti (made from 25 g wheat flour – atta)
Maida 25 g
Rice or rice flour 25 g
1 slice of bread
1 oz (30 g) noodles
Corn, bajra, jowar, 25 g

Substitution for 25 g pulses
25 g Lentil / beans / legumes (e.g. moong, channa, rajma, chole, kidney beans, peas)
Fish 100 g

Substitution for 25 g pulses
Chicken 100 g
Meat 50 g
Paneer 50 g (not fried)
Tofu 100 g

Equivalents for 200 g vegetables
Equal quantity of salads, including lettuce, cabbage, cucumber, tomato, onion
Equal quantity of green leafy vegetables
100 g potato, yam or sweet potato
Note: Count green peas under pulses, not vegetables

Equivalent of 1 fruit
1 fruit = 1 apple, orange, guava, pear, custard apple (sita phal), chikku, pomegranate
15 strawberries
15 grapes
20 cherries
1 ½ cup watermelon or 1 cup other melons
½ banana
½ mango

Equivalent of ½ scoop protein shake
½ scoop Isopure (or other brands) of protein shake (about 12 g protein and 100 calories in ½ scoop)
Egg whites 2 to 3
½ protein bar such as Quest Protein bar (about 11 g protein and 100 cal in ½ bar)

Options for fun stuff
1 small scoop ice cream (e.g. single-serving cup of Amul ice cream)
Chocolate 20 g (e.g. half a 45 g Cadbury Dairy Milk bar)
3 chocolate-dipped strawberries
2 macaroon cookies
1 cup jelly
1 piece rasgulla
One 20 g piece pista or kaju barfi

What About Alcohol?

Okay. The next question from some of you: what about alcohol? Well, alcohol has calories. For those who wish to calculate themselves, alcohol has 7 calories per gram. So, consider a wine that has 10 per cent alcohol. One hundred mL of this wine will have 10 mL alcohol (10 per cent), which will be 10 x 7 = 70 calories. While it will depend on alcohol percentage, typically, a glass of wine (about 150 mL) will have around 120 calories, a 30-mL peg of whisky will have 70 calories and a bottle of beer (about 360 mL) will have 140 calories (about 100 calories in a light beer). These amounts can vary based on the brand and the amount of alcohol. However, as a rule of thumb, to compensate for the calories in one alcoholic drink, you will have to eat at least a fruit less or one less roti or a bread slice next day. You could also try increasing your walk by 1.6 kilometre (or 1 mile) the next day, over and above the regular activity. And, all this is to (somewhat) compensate for the calories in one drink. Of course, you do miss out on nutrients if you eat a fruit less to compensate. It becomes really hard to compensate for calories in case of heavy drinking and I would neither recommend heavy drinking, nor compensating too much. It would be hard to get adequate calories and nutrients in a day, if the compensation for three or more drinks is attempted from a diet that is already lower in calories for weight loss. Hence, do not compensate for drinks over two in a day. In case you take more than two drinks a day, just accept a compromise that your weight loss will be somewhat slower.

An often-recognized issue with weight loss and alcohol is the 'munchies' that we eat with drinks. Drinks are mostly enjoyed in a social setting, maybe an evening with friends and family. Can you think what else you see in this picture along with alcohol? Masala nuts, cashews, bhajiya, bhujiya, paneer or chicken kababs, fried papad and more. About seven cashews or half a fried papad is calorically equal to one peg of whisky. We may know the number of drinks we had, but have you counted the number of nuts or bhajiya you ate during that time? The point being that substantial amounts of calories will go unnoticed when munchies are eaten with alcoholic drinks. A better way is to keep track of the accompanying snacks you are eating. We will address this in detail in a subsequent chapter.

What is 'free'?

There are a few items that have no or low calories and could be consumed within reasonable limits, without the fear of throwing your diet off. Water, black tea or coffee do not have calories. Same is true with diet drinks such as diet Coke, Coke Zero and diet Pepsi. Coconut water (not the malai), buttermilk or lassi (made from a sweetener) or clear soups have very few calories. Calories in spices (masala used for cooking) can vary, depending on the ingredients. However, considering the small amount used for cooking, one does not need to worry about the calories in spices. Some other examples of food that have calories, but could be considered as negligible due to the small amount we consume, include paan (beetle leaf), supari (beetle nut), or similar condiments. Sugar-free chewing gum has no calories. Also, some people love to eat mint or a small hard candy (orange or strawberry flavoured sweets) after meals. These are also okay when eaten just a couple or so a day. Another approach to lower calorie intake is to use cooking oil sprays such as the Pam spray to cook instead of deep frying.

Preventing Diet Boredom with Creative Cooking

You will notice that the Table 5 and 6 recommend food categories, but not specific food preparation. This is done intentionally to allow more freedom, flexibility and variety in diet. For instance, you could have vegetables of your choice under the 'vegetable' category, or change from roti, to naan, to phulka, to any other bread preparations, using the recommended amount of flour. I have noticed that my patients who were creative with their food preparation avoided boredom and had more success with their weight loss. The following are just a few examples to unlock your own creativity with food preparations.

A popular way to combine milk products and fruits for patients that have a sweet tooth is making ice cream or milk shakes from the prescribed amount of milk and fruit with a sugar substitute such as Splenda. Milkshakes can be a filling snack or dessert, since they are high volume and fill up the stomach. A different way to prepare fruit, rather than eating it plain, is to prepare fruit chaat. Chaat is also an excellent way to prepare pulses, such as channa. Just as there are many possible preparations with wheat flour, rice may be taken in many ways to add variety to the diet. It could be taken as pulao prepared with some of the vegetables, or even made into dosa. Or, puffed rice can be made at home for bhel puri preparations.

Lower calorie diets, such as those we prescribe, are often rich in fruits and vegetables to ensure adequate vitamin and mineral intake without exceeding calorie limits. Vegetables do not have to be taken as cooked vegetables, but can be combined with fruit, spices, salt, sugar, coriander and lime or lemon to make salads. Boiled pulses such as moong or channa also make excellent addition to such salads and side dishes to add variety, and don't always need to be used as daal.

Many meat preparations are also possible within the context of a low-calorie diet. Preparations with a lot of cream or ghee should be avoided, but tandoori preparations, marinated with yogurt and spices, are a good option. Kebabs can usually be made by marinating and roasting in the oven or on a grill with very little oil. Finally, roasted preparations can be eaten with rice or roti, but can also be made into a 'Frankie' or sandwich by using some of the prescribed wheat flour for making bread or chapati.

SUMMARY

- Note the ten components of a healthful diet for weight loss. A healthful diet considers many aspects of nutrition and not just calories. Not only what you eat, but even the timing in a day especially for foods that provide protein is important.
- Diet selection: Select a diet with calorie level that matches your need.
- Consider options and substitutions: Several options and choices are provided. Mix and match as desired. Such changes keep diets interesting and avoid monotony.
- Alcohol and weight loss diet: Alcohol has substantial calories. Also, be aware that the snacks eaten with alcohol

sometimes give more calories than alcohol itself. It is possible to compensate for the calories in alcohol only to a certain extent.

- Compensation: Best thing is to have no 'cheat days'. The next best is to compensate to some extent next day.

- Be creative: The diet is intentionally designed to give maximum flexibility and freedom. Use creativity to prepare various dishes and combinations from the basic ingredients recommended. This variation will contribute to your weight loss success.

- More resources: You can find more recipes, diet plans, and instructions at our website at: www.dhurandhar.com

5

Aamir Khan's Perfect Dangal

In June 2015, I met someone who would prove to be one of my most challenging patients ever. A patient with a nearly impossible goal. Mr Aamir Khan told me about a movie he was shooting – *Dangal*, the true story of wrestling legend Mahavir Singh Phogat. For the first part of his shoot, he had gained a lot of fat to portray the 'old Mahavir'. Now, for the second part he had to lose this gained fat, and more, to play a chiselled 'young Mahavir.' Providing guidance to lose fat is what I do, and indeed have done for thousands of patients. His next request, however, was an extraordinary challenge.

To be at his most muscular, Aamir Khan needed to not only lose multiple kilos of fat, he had to simultaneously gain several kilos of muscle. This is physiologically very difficult. The body loses weight (either fat and/or muscle) if it has less food than it requires in a day (also known as dieting). The body gains weight (fat and/or muscle) only if it has more food than it requires. In other words, muscle loss occurs during food deficit and muscle gain requires conditions of food surplus. How can the two happen at once? More so, I had only worked with patients – especially with challenging requests – in person. How was I supposed to treat a jetsetter like Aamir Khan, who was halfway around the world?

I looked back on my thirty years of experience as an obesity researcher, and the 15,000 patients I had treated for obesity as a physician, and decided to use a very specific, highly calibrated protein-powered diet. For a dedicated dieter, this works stunningly well, and Aamir is an extraordinarily disciplined and capable individual. Through his efforts, those of his exercise trainers and my guidance, the diet worked. He lost approximately 17 kg weight, including 13 kg of fat and gained a net 2 kg of muscle (and even more gross muscle gain). He reached the desired goal of having less than 10 per cent body fat for shooting. Successfully treating Aamir from nearly 15,000 km away encouraged me to share a version of this diet to help others. That was the genesis of this book.

I should mention that my father, Dr Vinod Dhurandhar and I have treated people for obesity who come from all walks of life and occupations. This includes celebrities from different fields, politicians, prominent leaders or professionals, or individuals from the film industry. One thing we are extremely careful about is honouring the doctor–patient relationship and protecting the patient's privacy. Hence, we have always been tight-lipped about our patients, and have never used the names of our high-profile patients to get publicity or attention for us. Aamir Khan would have been no exception and he would have gone without any mention by me. However, it was Aamir who publicly announced my name as his nutritionist for *Dangal*, and the floodgates of inquiry opened. Before starting to respond to all media and personal inquiries, I contacted Aamir. I mentioned that now that he was repeatedly mentioning my name, I will have to respond to the inquiries. What aspects of his treatment could I divulge? His response was: 'Tell them everything.' He did not want to hold back any aspects of the treatment. So, here is the story:

My first meeting with Aamir was going to be at his place in Bandra. I was visiting India at the time and did not have a clinic where we could meet. He sent a car for me, so finding the place was not my concern. I made my way through numerous security personnel and I was finally ushered into a drawing room. Four men greeted me. I scanned the group, but absolutely could not recognize Aamir. Was I in the right place? Finally, a heavy-set man with comforting smile and piercing eyes extended the arm to shake hands. We connected!

So, here was the plan: In preparation for the movie, he had been gaining muscle to get the appearance and strength of a wrestler and had also intentionally gained weight to portray the older Mahavir Phogat. When that shooting was completed, he wanted to lose the excess fat to make the muscle underneath visible and to also gain additional muscle to look like the younger wrestling champion. This phase was going to end on 10 June 2016. And, my job was to help him reach below 10 per cent body fat by that deadline. In subsequent interactions, I had such a renewed respect for the efforts that went in getting Aamir ready for the role. His workouts varied during the time, but often started at 4 a.m. and included cardio training for 45 minutes, serious weight training for 75 minutes, wrestling lessons, walking and running. At times, he was spending 6–7 hours a day exercising. I promptly decided to depend on the physical trainer for his activity and focused on addressing his nutritional needs. I also requested his family doctor to be aware of the programme we were initiating and received his input and approval. I was in the US and Aamir was in Mumbai. Both of us travelled a lot. But, we FaceTimed every week, or at times several times a week and used emails and WhatsApp for regular communication.

With Aamir's input, I proposed a combination of diets that would match his phase of workouts. For some periods, his workouts were mainly focused on burning calories, and other times they would promote body building. During the calorie burning times, he would have a diet of about 1,800 calories and during the body building times, the diet calories were increased to 2,100–2,300 per day. These diets were designed to provide about 100–110 g protein per day. These were not 'very high protein' diets. I advised him to break down the diet in small and frequent meals, about six meals a day.

And, then I ran into my first challenge

Here is the WhatsApp message from Aamir that posed the challenge:

AK: I have been thinking a lot about the diet
and I have concluded that I would really like to
try a vegan diet. I know, I should have told you
earlier.... No eggs, no milk products, no dairy.

Okay. He wanted to bulk up and build significant muscles,
while losing fat simultaneously. Not an easy task on a regular
vegetarian diet, but doable. This is because vegetarian foods
contain more calories for a given amount of protein. For
example, 25 g protein can be obtained from fish or chicken,
daals, or milk. But the calories in a fish/chicken portion that
provides 25 g protein would be about 100. Whereas, daals and
milk (even if skimmed milk) will give 300 to 350 calories to
provide 25 g protein. Moreover, as a vegan, he did not even
want milk, except in tea. So, now my job was to come up with
a diet that excluded milk and dairy products, eggs and all meats,
and the one that was lower in calories and higher in protein.
An interesting challenge that I overcame.

Aamir was very meticulous about reporting what he ate
daily. Here is one of his early reports:

6 a.m.

Protein shake (30 g)

7.15 a.m.

Upma 50 g with 100 g tomato and onions, coriander and
chilly (not measured) cooked with 1 teaspoon oil

1 cup tea with little milk

9.30 a.m.
   2 cups of tea with little milk

12.30 p.m.
   Pineapple 100 g
   1 vegan protein bar

2.00 p.m.
   Vegetables 250 g
   Rotis 2 (25 g wheat flour, each)
   Dal 50 g
   Rice 50 g

4.30 p.m.
   Nuts 50 g
   Raisins 30 g

6.30 p.m.
   Melon 200 g

10.00 p.m.
   Vegetables 250 g
   Bread 4 slices
   Dal 50 g
   Rice 50 g

All foods cooked in a total of 5 teaspoon of oil.

He was eating eight meals a day. Better than my advice of eating six meals a day. Well begun is half done. At least, so I thought at the time. Just then we ran into another bump in the road. He was unable to consistently adhere to the diet. There were temptations, social events and other reasons occasionally throwing the diet off. This was completely understandable, especially considering his recent diet history. He just had a long period of weight gain for the movie role, in which he had gained about 27 kg by eating indiscriminately. By his own admission, he was eating just about everything to gain weight. And, now, suddenly he was trying to press the brake. I knew that his body would take some time to turn around from the weight gain mode to the weight loss mindset. The perfectionist in him, however, was unable to come to terms with it. Here is a message from him that speaks volumes:

> AK: Dr Nikhil, I'm afraid this week has not gone well either ☹ I have broken the diet so many times this week that I feel embarrassed to report to you. I'm sorry, I feel I'm letting you down. And, of course, in the process I'm letting myself down too. I seem to be having trouble being strict with myself. Please help me.

And, my self-explanatory response to him:

> ND: Of course, that is my role. There is ABSOLUTELY NOTHING to be embarrassed

about. I should know better than anyone that weight loss is not easy to achieve. If it were easy, we would not need professional help. Moving on: 1) Please send your weight; 2) Do not give up diet because you had a lapse or two. Those are battles, not the war; 3) Let's talk and review what you need at this time; 4) Call me tomorrow your time, 8 a.m.

He persevered. Hats off to his resilience. Then came the times he was travelling abroad and needed diets for the countries he was visiting. I loved creating these diets for him – he promised to follow them even when travelling, and kept his promise. Soon, he was back on track. Texts were coming in expressing his satisfaction with adherence to diet. Any change would get reported too. Here is an example:

AK: Morning Doc. Last night, there were some guests over for dinner, and I ate dahi and two pakoras, which are not a part of my diet. And, two spoons dessert. Rest I stuck to my diet.

I wish I had all patients reporting so candidly. The time passed quickly and he had lost 5 kg or so. Long way to go. During these times of frequent FaceTime calls, our conversations drifted to many other topics. Although both of us were perpetually pressed for time, I very much enjoyed our little detours in conversations. For example, a discussion about the accent used in the movie *Dangal* led to him telling me about various Indian languages and how they may differ slightly in saying the same word, or how geography influences languages. He mentioned that in cold countries, warm is considered pleasing and vice versa. For instance, a loving heart is considered 'warm' in western culture and 'cool' in Indian culture. On other occasions, we talked about his campaign to address famine once and for all in Maharashtra and we exchanged views about the recent books we have read. What absolutely floored me was to hear from him the meaning of '*Pasaydaan*', in the final chapter of '*Dnyaneshwari, a Treatise on Bhagvad Gita*'. It was a wonderful exchange. During the time, my understanding of him went from Aamir Khan as a patient to Aamir Khan as a brilliant, well-read person with deep understanding of several topics, a person with great discipline and laser sharp focus. This understanding was to come very handy during the time that lay ahead and which was going to test both of us.

Towards the end of 2015, he was around 94 kg and near 30 per cent body fat. His firm requirement was 10 per cent body fat, and huge muscles, and the firm deadline was still 10 June 2016. I was worried about meeting the deadline and tried negotiating the deadline, in case he needed more time. No such luck. The deadline was immovable. Five months to lose 20 per cent body fat and 14 to 15 kg weight. Three kg per month loss for five straight months. It was probably doable, at least in theory. But, we could not afford any setbacks. How I wished I had a magic wand. There was none. So, I got to work. We divided the five months in four phases. Phase 1: Muscle gain. Phase 2: Weight loss. Phase 3: Muscle building and Phase 4, the final phase: Fat loss. Gain in muscle in each phase was going to help the weight or fat loss phase that followed.

Phase 1 started very well. In the first four weeks of the new year's diet, he knocked off 4 kg, despite an elbow injury. But, Aamir was ever vigilant. He wrote:

> AK: Last week, I did not train, as my elbow has been troubling me. So, I wanted to rest it for a week. So, I dropped one meal post workout. Since I did not workout, I dropped that meal. Tomorrow, I will be back to my workout.

It was now time to activate my master plan for Phase 2. By now, I knew his resolve. But, I also had come to recognize the events that would interfere with our plan. I proposed that Aamir should be sequestered from India, come to the US for three to four weeks and stay secluded at a resort. Here, away from his social and other commitments, he would focus only on his diet and activity. That's it. No other distractions. I was confident that this would help. Aamir agreed, with one condition – he wanted to follow my diet at the resort. I got to work and started calling various resorts to identify one that would fit our plan, and allow Indian diet that I planned for him. After a search, I found the right place for him.

This was a resort away from city life, tucked away in the mountains of the American west. It catered to select people who were interested in improving health in various ways. Aamir was there for three weeks, walking, biking, swimming, hiking, and building muscle six to seven hours a week. We estimated that he was burning about 1,500 to 1,800 calories a day just exercising. Just for perspective, you will need to walk about 30 km/day to burn 1,800 calories a day. We increased his diet to about 2,300 calories per day and the protein amount, so that he would not experience too large a calorie deficit. I was specifically careful about hydration in the desert. He would lose a large amount of water and body salts due to sweat. It was important to recover those salts along with water. The result of this hard work? Six kg lost in three weeks. This was fantastic. Ten kg down. Aamir was also happy. He wrote:

AK: Thank you, Doc. I'm heading back to India today. Thank you for the great suggestion of this resort. It really gave me the boost I needed, and it has inspired me to go forward from here.

At this time, the hype around Aamir's weight loss started building in India. Reporters discovered that he was out of India for weight loss. Expectations around his weight loss for *Dangal* were skyrocketing. No pressure for me, of course! There was no time to waste. Phases 3 and 4 were to follow. As planned, there was not much weight loss anticipated in

Phase 3. Only muscle building. Overall, it went OK, with a flurry of phone calls and back and forth of questions and suggestions. Day after day after day, Aamir was resisting temptations and working away in the gym. Five weeks before the shooting was to begin, his weight had gone up a bit, but he body fat had dropped down to 15 per cent. Five more per cent of fat to lose. The slight bump in body weight was clearly due to the muscle build-up. And, I got this message:

> AK: I am afraid last week was not good. The travel was very bad for my diet. My routine broke and I ended up eating stuff.

It was going to be now or never. I got on a call with Aamir. We chatted. It was time to move to Phase 4 and focus on fat loss. It was going to be on a 1,500-calorie diet. Two weeks remaining and his fat was at 14 per cent. And, after that call, things went silent. There was no contact from Aamir. No reports, no queries, no texts. Nothing. I knew he must be busy preparing for the shoot. One day, I got the following message:

> AK: 19 June 2016: Good morning doctor. I have good news. I am at the shoot in Ludhiana, shooting for the scenes for which I needed to get back into shape. My body fat is 10.08 per cent. Visually, my body is looking very good. We have

reached our goal! Thank you. It was wonderful working with you.

My immediate response:

ND: This is SUPERB! I am very impressed. You were an absolutely outstanding patient with keen understanding and a terrific determination. For my part, I feel good to have delivered. All the very best!

Here is what Aamir Khan had achieved with great determination and struggle. It was not easy at all, but now it was an example for many.

Table 7: Aamir's achievement

	July 2015	June 2016
Body Weight (kg)	96.7	80
Fat per cent	38.3	10.08
Chest (inches)	44.5	43
Waist (inches)	43	32
Hips (inches)	44	39

6

Exercise Is a Supplement, Not a Substitute

Exercise has a tonne of health benefits for both body and mind. However, it may surprise you to learn that *exercise is not needed for weight loss*. One can lose weight with diet alone. But it doesn't work the other way. In fact, it is nearly impossible to lose weight with exercise alone, without paying attention to diet. Stay with me and allow me to explain.

Broadly speaking, the physical benefits of exercise could be divided in three categories: 1) burning calories; 2) increasing lung capacity and improving cardiovascular system; and 3) building or preserving muscle. Although all types of exercises will provide the benefit of burning calories, and there will be some overlap in benefits, the other two benefits depend on the type of activity or exercise. Activities such as running, swimming, cardio training, skipping rope, will mainly increase stamina, improve lung and heart capacity. Whereas, exercises involving weight lifting will mainly build muscle mass. Now, which of these exercises should you choose while you are following a weight-loss diet? Should you join a gym? Take up a sport? Dance lessons? Yoga?

Avoid these exercises: Let's first see what is *not* a good exercise for many struggling with extra weight. One very important principle to recognize during dieting is to ensure no harm comes because of exercise. When you have serious weight issues, joints such as back, lower back, hip or knee are already carrying more load than what they are designed for. The same is true with most other body systems. Your lungs, heart, liver, are overworking due to the excess load the body is carrying. Imagine what will happen to all these joints and organs if you start skipping a jump rope when you are a 120 kg man or say 80 kg woman of average height? Or, if you start running, lifting heavy weights or suddenly decide to go mountain climbing? You are likely to invite trouble. It is better to stay away from these exercises or very strenuous activities such as fast bicycling, singles tennis or badminton, or basketball, that will tax your body systems while you are very heavy. There will be a time to engage in these activities. That would be after you lose weight. If you feel very strongly about engaging in such vigorous activities, consult your doctor for an opinion.

Consider these exercises: Now, let's see what exercise may be compatible with weight loss. During a diet, you need exercise to burn calories and to preserve the muscle mass. Calories burned due to exercise contribute to the energy deficit that you are creating with diet and they help lose fat. Also, remember that calories are mainly burnt by our muscles. Bigger the muscle, greater is the burning of calories, and better the fat loss. During weight loss, we tend to lose some muscle, no matter how well-planned and well-executed your diet may be. So, if our muscle decreases, we burn fewer calories. This makes it harder to lose weight further and makes it easier to regain. Therefore, it is very important to minimize muscle loss during weight loss. Exercise is a way to strengthen muscles and minimize their loss during dieting.

Here, let me make an extremely important point, especially for women. I see that many women switch off their mind the moment they hear the word 'muscles'. It is their belief that muscles are for men, not women. Wrong. All humans have muscles, men as well as women. Just like both men and women have bones but in differing sizes, the size of muscles is bigger in men compared to women. Muscles play the same role of body movement and calorie burning in men and women. So, it is equally important for both to exercise during weight loss and preserve muscle. Preserving muscles is not the same as building more muscles like a bodybuilder. That type of muscle-building needs a different type of heavy exercise, which is not the intent of the exercise needed during weight loss.

The best exercise: The best exercise you can do during weight-loss period is the one that causes no harm, burns some calories and helps preserve the muscle mass. An example of such exercise is slow and level walking. Not brisk walking or jogging, and not climbing up and down stairs. Just good old level walking. Level walking ensures that you are not unduly taxing your heart or back. In fact, the calf muscles are called our 'second heart', which pump blood back to heart when walking and thus helping the circulatory system.

Walking involves big muscles in the body (thigh, leg and back muscles), which use substantial number of calories. They help you meet the goals of burning calories and preserving muscle mass. Now, about the 'slow walking' part. It is a principle of physics that if the distance is constant, whether you walk, run or jog, the calories burned will be nearly identical. According to the formula, work done = force x distance; or if simplified a bit, it translates to calories burned = body weight x distance. As you can see, there is no place to include speed or duration in this formula. To slowly walk three kilometres, you will need about 40 minutes and you will burn about 160-200 calories in the process. If you run the same distance, you may cover the distance in perhaps 20 minutes, but still burn about the same calories. Why, then, would you run that distance while carrying several excess kilos of body weight and run the risk of hurting yourself?

Another consideration is that if you are running, you are likely to be out of breath in a kilometre and a half or so, having consumed 80–100 calories, and may not run any further. Whereas, if you are walking at a leisurely pace, you may cover 3, or even 4, kilometres without running out of steam, and receive additional calorie benefits. Therefore, slow and level walking is the best exercise under the given circumstances for people struggling to lose excess weight.

Some people are unable to walk temporarily or permanently due to some physical ailment. They may use a wheel chair for mobility. Many of them experience body weight struggles. In this situation, if one cannot walk, perhaps consider any activity involving shoulder movements, if possible. Shoulder muscles are not as big as thigh muscles. Hence, the benefit of activity involving shoulder muscles will be lesser than that due to walking. Nonetheless, in this case something is better than nothing.

The second-best exercise: The next best exercise to walking is swimming or water aerobics (water-based exercise), if you have the facility. Swimming involves many big muscles in the body and burns calories. It gives a nice workout to the whole body and gets your heart pumping too. Also, the buoyancy of water eases pressure on the weight bearing joints. So, those who are unable to walk due to joint pains find swimming or water-based exercise helpful. There are also some reasons why swimming is the second, not the first, on my list. In addition to other benefits, walking also strengthens bones, swimming does not. Also, unlike walking, swimming requires access to a pool, special clothing and convenience logistics to be addressed. At times, it may take you 30 minutes each way to commute to and from the pool. You may not have that much time. Also, people tend to count the minutes they were in the pool as calories burned. However, the time that you sat in the pool chatting with your friend does not count. So, the net time you actually burn calories by swimming may be far less than what you think. Instead, walking can be undertaken more easily and in many locations. Nonetheless, if swimming is what you prefer and enjoy, so be it.

Developing a walking programme: As you start the weight loss diet, support it with the right type and amount of exercise and ensure that the programme is not short lived. I highly recommend slow and level walking, over other activities for this purpose. This is doable for most anyone, does not require fancy equipment or place, easy on your joints and body and not unpleasant, hence, sustainable. Here are some key aspects that you may wish to consider in developing such a walking programme.

Get ready: There is some basic preparation even for your walking programme to ensure success and sustainability.

- Decide on a time and a place to walk. If you have not been walking for exercise, aim for 30 minutes a day. Now, here is a secret. You don't need 30 minutes at a stretch. You could walk for 10 minutes, three times, or even 5 minutes at a time, six times a day. Where you walk is important for sustainability. If your walk involves a 45 minute drive to a joggers park, rest assured that you will follow this for only the initial week or so while your enthusiasm lasts. Find a place that is convenient for every day. It could be a combination of your road, backyard, terrace, office hallways or even your own house or bedroom. No need to wait to find THE perfect spot or the perfect day to start. Just start!

- Enlist a friend, neighbour or family member to walk with you. This social interaction keeps you company, gives something to look forward to and makes walking interesting. Also, your friend will motivate you on days when you feel like skipping the daily walk and the sense of commitment keeps you going (in turn, you also influence your friend similarly). Beware, however, that it could also go in the opposite direction. You may be ready for your walk and your friend cancels on you. Don't let that impact your resolve. After all, it is your health and you need to be in charge of it. Walking with friends works for many, but not all. Choose what suits you best.

- When it comes to walking, your initial enthusiasm is your best friend. But, this friendship may not last long. Yet, you need to keep the walking programme going, even after the enthusiasm fades. There are some barriers that you could reduce and stick to this regimen till it becomes second nature. You are likely to avoid an activity that is unpleasant. If walking is too strenuous or painful, you are less likely to bring upon yourself a punishment day after day. Keep it simple.

The other thing that works for me is to keep my gear ready. I get ready for my exercise first thing in the morning and keep my exercise clothes and shoes ready at night, and directly jump into those shoes in the morning. This is even on my off days. If too bored, I promise myself that let me just wear the shoes. After that if I don't feel like working out, I will take that day off. Magic happens after I wear those shoes. Most of the times, after having overcome the initial boredom and inertia, I rarely not work out. Try it.

- A final recommendation in your preparation is to have some way to measure your workout to monitor progress. In this case, to be able to count your steps. The most inexpensive way is to simply count the steps for the distance you will be walking. At my height (5'10"), I need about 2,000 foot steps to complete 1 mile or 1.6 kilometres. A taller person may need somewhat fewer steps and a shorter person may need more steps to cover the same distance. The range would probably be 1,800-2,200 steps, depending on your height. If you are walking on the terrace of your building or even in your house, count the footsteps that one round makes and then simply keep track of how many rounds you took.

A somewhat more sophisticated approach is to use your smart phone to count the steps. Many smart phones have apps that can easily do this. Obviously, the smart phone needs to be on you. But, you may not carry it on you throughout the day. This can provide only a part snapshot of daily activity. There are also the pedometers which are fairly inexpensive. Be careful about correct placement of the pedometers that you tuck into clothes at your waist so that they can track steps accurately. In my experience, many of them need to be placed over to the far side, away from the umbilicus, to give accurate readings. Many are not very convenient and accurate for women wearing sarees.

A recent option that is slightly more expensive, but much more accurate and convenient is the pedometers to wear on the wrist. They look like wrist watches and give you time, number of steps or distance walked, and even the duration and quality of sleep. The one that I wear is waterproof and does not need to be removed during a bath or swimming. I wear it round the clock, so it captures the entire day's activity, not only when I decide to go for a walk or a run. A device, such as what I wear, is a great motivator. A glance at it during the day tells how my day is going, walking-wise. I can step up my efforts, if needed, to meet my day's goal. This wrist-pedometer has become like a personal trainer, monitoring my walking and motivating me to walk more.

Two-week plan: I know of many people who have been fired up to start exercise and take on way more than they can handle on the very first day. They then stay in bed for the next week because of a pulled muscle or back pain. Starting gradually and easing into a routine is the key to avoid such situations. Here is a way to establish your walking plan over a period of two weeks.

- Note your baseline and increase gradually: A good goal is to complete 10,000 steps in a day, that includes walking for your daily activity, plus the exercise. First, it is important to note the number of steps you are currently taking. If you are around 3,000-4,000 steps a day, do not start with 10,000 steps the next day. Increase by 500 steps a day. So, start with 3,000 steps today, make them 3,500 tomorrow, and 4,000 the day after, so you should be able to add 7,000 more steps in two weeks or so. If this transition is also too rapid, take it easy and increase by 500 steps every other day.

  If you are already taking say 8,000 steps a day before starting this programme, then going up to 10,000 steps should not be hard for you. But, in that case instead of a goal of 10,000 steps, consider a higher number of steps as your eventual goal. The point is to increase physical activity over and beyond the current level.

- If possible, spread your exercise over the course of the day in two or more sessions. This allows you to go easy when you are just starting out. More importantly, you are also distributing your risk of missing exercise. If you exercise every day at 8 a.m. only and something makes you miss this slot, then you have missed your scheduled exercise till next day. Instead, if you walk a bit at 8 a.m. and then again at 6 p.m., you still have the other time slot to get at least some steps done. Something is better than nothing.

• Consider it 'non-negotiable' to meet your target of steps for a day. Only then will you start finding ways to meet your goal. Here is what I did just today. It was a Saturday and I had taken my car for a wash. You hand over the car to those folks, who clean the interior of the car first, then send it through a big, long moving belt where the machine washes the car automatically, and then the folks there dry it and hand it back to you. Today, I needed a real thorough and deep cleaning of the exterior and the interior, which was going to take 45 minutes. They have a lovely waiting room where people sit, watch TV or watch through a glass wall how the car wash machine is cleaning their cars. Instead of sitting down or standing for 45 minutes like other customers there, I chose a secluded hallway and at a slow pace I walked up and down while reading emails on my phone. It took them 50 minutes to clean my car and I got 5,000 steps done in that time. That was a bonus. Just walk where and when you get a chance.

Admittedly, in big cities like Mumbai, car parking is a big issue. But, this seems to be compounded by our insistence on finding parking directly in front of the shop, store, or a restaurant that we are visiting. If at times we are willing to add 5 to 7 minutes walking, parking may be available and you get extra steps. It is worth mentioning a research concept here. The concept is that you compare the total daily physical activity of two groups of people. Those who exercise daily at a designated time versus those who did not have any structured exercise in their day. Surprisingly, both groups will have similar total daily physical activity. It turns out that those who specifically exercise, may take the rest of the day easy and do not care to walk the rest of the time as if they had met the activity quota for the day. On the other hand, those who do not have designated time for exercise perhaps feel guilty about it and they try to compensate for it by at least parking cars a bit far, or taking the stairs instead of taking the lift and try adding some activity. A message for us? Don't be sedentary throughout the rest of the day just because you got your morning (or evening) session of exercise done. Every little bit of walking counts.

- The concept of 'rest days' does not apply to this exercise. Rest days are for high intensity workouts that allow heavily worked muscles to rest and recover, while you focus on different types of muscle groups. Slow and level walking of up to 10,000 steps a day is such a gentle exercise that your muscles don't need much recovery. Your body is working every day and needs the benefits of this exercise daily. So, no rest days.

Keep it going: To start an exercise plan is relatively easy compared to continuing it. There are some landmines to navigate that can bring your programme down. Here are some of them and what to do to overcome those challenges. Forewarned is forearmed.

- A point related to 'no rest days': while we need exercise every day, it is possible that on some days or on a series of days it may just not be possible to exercise. First, the focus should be on minimizing such no-workout days. But, if it does happen, remember the words: Lapse, relapse, collapse. Missing exercise occasionally on a day or a couple of days is a lapse, a temporary deviation from your routine. Just get back on your schedule at the first chance you get instead of lamenting about the lapse, blaming yourself for lack of discipline and so on, which can lead to a relapse, a prolonged break from exercise. This could lead to complete collapse of the entire workout programme.

- Success can hurt. Too many pats on the back from friends and family who are complimenting on your dieting and weight loss can be heady and have a disarming effect. The urge to continue exercise starts diminishing bit by bit. Feeling accomplished is good, losing weight and feeling physically fit is a great feeling, but it is not something you deposit in the bank and earn an interest on, lifelong. You have to earn this feeling every day. So, no stopping.

- It's not only about weight loss. Exercise helps us in so many ways. Exercise should be a way of life, regardless of weight loss. Don't stop it after you reach your goal weight. In fact, as we will see in subsequent chapters, exercise becomes even more important during your transition to weight maintenance phase. This long-term commitment to exercise is possible only if you have carefully chosen the type of activity as outlined above. You will stick to exercise, if you don't make it a punishment.

Exercise myths: Just like nutrition, exercise is a field of science. Scientific advice in both fields should come from those who have studied it. The Internet is not necessarily the best place to get information about nutrition or exercise, unless it comes from qualified authorities. There are many misconceptions and notions that can mislead you. It is important to know the facts. Here are some common myths related to exercise that can mislead you and interfere with your exercise programme.

a. *Sweating is needed to burn calories*: Not true. Sweating is a way for the body to cool down when overheated. Some people sweat a lot and some sweat little. It is not an indication of how many calories you burned. So, don't be disappointed if you walk but don't sweat. What's more, sweating itself by taking sauna bath or steam bath is not connected with any fat loss. So, if you have the time, use it for walking and not sitting in a sauna hoping to lose fat.

b. *Massage increases weight loss*: Getting a massage improves circulation and that feels great. But, it has no effect on fat loss. Nor can you displace your fat with massage from one body part to other. The human body is not a tube of toothpaste.

c. *Twist your waist to reduce it*: Exercise has no effect on local fat. If you bend a few times, your abdominal muscle could firm up. But, that action of bending has not much effect on fat stored on your abdomen. When it comes to losing fat in response to diet and exercise, the body has a mind of its own. We cannot control the sequence or the amount of fat loss from each fat depot. A point to note: when carrying excess weight, wrong or excessive bending could contribute to problems of spine such as a slipped disc.

d. *Women should avoid exercise as they will get bulky muscles*: Yes and no. Women can get bigger muscles if they do exercises that build muscles, such as heavy weight lifting. Slow, level walking is not designed to build muscles, but to burn calories and to prevent muscle loss. Neither men nor women will 'build big muscles' from slow and level walking as described above.

e. *Exercise is not needed once you become thin*: False. Exercise is needed for almost everyone, regardless of weight. Slim or otherwise. Even slim people benefit from exercise. When you lose weight, it becomes even more important to keep burning calories regularly to help maintain weight loss. Make it a part of your daily routine like bathing or brushing teeth. Research studies have shown that those who exercise regularly have much better success with maintaining the weight lost.

f. *No pain no gain:* The thought that you need to exercise till it hurts is a dangerous one, especially for people struggling with weight. The type of activity, duration and severity should be such that there is no pain. For one thing, you are not likely to continue a painful activity on a long-term basis. So, if something is hurting, stop and take rest, or seek medical advice as appropriate.

Some Common Questions

1. Should I use a stationary bike?

   Your choice. Unlike skipping rope or running, a stationary bike may not put undue weight on your weight-bearing joints or tax the heart, if used in moderation, and yet burn some calories. However, if you have bad knees or bad back, this may not be best for you.

2. Do I need a personal exercise trainer?

   You don't need one especially if you are going to be walking. That said, good exercise trainers can be excellent coaches, motivators and counsellors if you are embarking on a training programme. They can also guide you appropriately to work out while minimizing the risk of injury. On the other hand, some exercise trainers also advise about nutrition, herbal and other supplements and food products, without much or any formal training or education in nutrition. I have heard some jaw-dropping nutritional advice and dangerous supplements recommended by some unscrupulous individuals. Frankly, it is your responsibility to seek the right guidance from the right person, based on their qualifications. For instance, I go to my dentist for my teeth. I would not seek advice from my dentist about my finances. Let nutritionists and exercise trainers do their separate jobs.

3. Should I walk before or after food?

In the larger scheme of things, food in relation to exercise does not matter much. Just exercise when it is convenient. If walking is uncomfortable right after food, don't do so. There are some conveniently spread beliefs about so-called health drinks or foods. I have noticed rows of vendors selling foods and drinks of different kind outside various parks. I see people lining up to them after their walks in the park. While I absolutely understand that being the livelihood for a vendor, there is no particular health benefit of timing a drink or food with walking. In fact, I have also seen people take a few rounds of the park, which may burn 100 or 200 calories, and then pleased with their accomplishment, step outside to eat a good 500-calorie dose of bhel puri, pani-puri or ragda patties. Obviously, this approach will not be productive for weight loss.

4. Should I join a gym? Take up a sport? Join dance lessons? Yoga?

    It depends. High impact dancing may carry the same concerns as jumping or running. Your priority is to get your daily steps in. If you are following the diet, walk 10,000 steps a day. If you still have some extra time to learn or practise some low impact dancing or yoga, so be it. Or, if you wish to use a treadmill or an elliptical to walk in a gym, that's fine. Just make sure to follow expert guidance so no harm comes to you. While physical, mental and spiritual benefits have been ascribed to yoga, in the form it is commonly practised, yoga is not a strong source of physical activity for burning calories, unlike walking. Remember that burning calories without harm is the goal during your weight-loss phase. Once you have lowered the weight, you may consider more active, physically demanding activities. That would in fact help build your lung capacity and cardiovascular endurance at that time.

5. Modern life is not conducive to exercise. What is the remedy?

    That is correct. There are very few opportunities for physical activity and they are continually decreasing. Just for fun, think of all the physical activity stuff you used to do 10 or 20 years ago, but not anymore. Here is an example. When I was very young, when the telephone rang, one had to walk up to the phone to answer it. It was in one room in the house. Then, perhaps walk back to the family member for whom the call was, to inform about the call. Eventually, the cordless phones arrived on the scene. There were many cordless phones in the house, in different rooms. So, one did not have to walk all the way to one room that had the phone. Next came cell phones, and the rest is history.

I grew up in Vile Parle, Mumbai. From our house to the railway station is a 7-minute walk and everyone around walked to the station. If you were rushed or older, you took the bus. Then came the rikshaws and I wonder if even one person walks that distance anymore. The point is labour-saving devices are all over and have become an integral part of our life. Let's just accept the fact that they are here to stay. Don't hold your breath for a time when we all will be again heading to the jungle to chop firewood, light fire, hunt our food and cook. That indeed will use more calories, but that is not happening. Stop lamenting about it. You will have to do all your hunting between the refrigerator and the microwave. So, how does one get the needed activity within the framework of existing facts?

Well, it is possible to meet or exceed the quota of physical activity if there is a will. You can turn the labour-saving devices into advantages. Microwaves are not a curse, but a boon, if you consider the time they save. I spend a lot of time on cell phones in a day. I keep pacing up and down in the room when on phone (something I could not have done with the old fashioned phone with cords). At home, you could place a treadmill or exercise bike in front of the TV. So, you need not be idle while watching your favourite shows. You can even purchase a set of bicycle pedals that could be placed in front of you as a foot stool, and pedal away when you are comfortably seated on a sofa. Do use your car or other vehicle to reach office in time. But, during your eight or nine hours at the office, get up every hour and walk 2.5 minutes in one direction and then return. That would be 5 minutes walking every hour – over 3 kilometres in one day (equal to about 200 calories). These alternatives would be independent of monsoon, rain, heat or cold, or other festivals and festivities, which often seem to stump people who are looking for a right time and setting to start physical activity. If there a will, there is a way.

Summary

- Fat loss with exercise alone is not likely. Exercise is not a substitute for dieting, but a supplement.
- The best exercise during weight loss is the one that causes no harm, burns some calories and helps preserve muscle mass.
- Slow and level walking is that exercise. Time of the day, place, or speed does not matter.

- Measuring and monitoring progress is important. Keep a track of the steps you take. Increase the number gradually.
- Keep it easy, simple and pleasant. You are unlikely to continue an unpleasant or painful activity for a long time. Your long-term commitment is important.
- Keep walking throughout the day. Be creative about snatching few minutes to keep walking.
- Steer clear of misconceptions and myths. Get professional advice from qualified exercise trainers if needed.

Start today. Take just 100 steps right after you read this and just see the magic of that resolve.

7

What to Expect During Weight Loss?

When You Start the Diet

What should you expect, now that you have embarked on a weight loss diet? When your doctor prescribes you a course of antibiotics, you don't have much choice other than taking those antibiotics. And as long as you take those pills, you'll recover. Weight loss, on the other hand, is a complex process that requires your active participation. A good understanding of this mechanism prepares you well to navigate the path. Wrong assumptions and incomplete information may ruin your weight loss efforts. Here is what to expect as your weight loss journey begins – and in particular – what to do if weight loss stalls.

- **Your blood sugar, blood pressure and energy levels get a boost**: One of the first things you will notice as you begin dieting is hunger. Your diet is designed to reduce calories without making you feel deprived or hungry. In general, however, a sudden change in the number of calories eaten can make you miss food and keep you feeling a bit hungry. You may miss food or think about it the whole day. You will envy people who are not dieting. You may feel the urge to even stop dieting. Here is the important point: this feeling is almost universal, but it lasts only two to four days. Get past those days and you will get used to the diet and start feeling better. *In just a week or two, you should begin to feel more energetic.* If you were previously feeling sleepy, tired or plain lethargic during the day, after you start the diet, those feelings will reduce. Many start experiencing a sense of control and purposefulness. Many a time, this is linked to an improvement in the functioning of insulin, which starts making sugar available to your body cells. This change is quite remarkable and can happen even before you have lost substantial body weight. This phenomenon is also reported in bariatric surgery (weight-loss surgery) cases. Many people who undergo surgery for weight loss show marked improvement in insulin and glucose levels even before substantial weight loss has occurred. Another condition that may improve quickly, even before substantial weight loss, is high blood pressure. In some individuals, high blood pressure may improve rapidly after starting weight loss diet.

It is important to be aware of these responses of the body, particularly if you are on medication for lowering blood sugar or blood pressure. Your doctor may have to adjust the doses of these medications. For example, if you need blood pressure medication to keep it down and your weight loss diet also normalizes blood pressure, the dose of blood pressure medication may have to be reduced. Vigilance is needed, but consider these as first benefits of a weight-loss diet. If your blood sugar or blood pressure are normal and you are not on medication for lowering them, this should not be a concern for you. A well-planned diet should not lower your blood sugar or blood pressure much if it is already normal.

- **Less bloating**: Another change that happens fairly soon into the process is a decrease in abdominal discomfort, reduction in feeling bloated and gassy, a common complaint linked with excess weight. The feeling of heartburn after a meal should improve after starting this diet. If it does not, it may not be diet related and you may need to consult the doctor to rule out other possible causes including the acidity. The old adage that 'hurry, worry and curry cause acidity' may no longer be true. Eating less spicy may not relieve acidity. Recent Nobel Prize-winning research has shown that often it is a bacterial infection in stomach that causes acidity, which can be easily be treated by a dose of antibiotics by your doctor.

The mention of spicy food reminds me of something. Traditional spices such as red chilly power, black pepper, turmeric, cardamom, curry powder have very few calories, if any. Plus, the amount used is so little that they could be considered virtually calorie free. The same does not hold true if coconut is added to these spices. A tablespoon of grated coconut can add as many calories as a small scoop of ice cream. While you can certainly have the coconut-free spices without worrying about their calorie content, you may find food spicier as you start dieting. This is because you will be reducing the amount of cooking oil in diet food, which otherwise masks the spiciness. Consider reducing the spice in food, if needed.

- **Possible constipation**: Along with benefits, there are also some challenges of eating a reduced-calorie diet. Some people may experience constipation. This is because the amount of food that you were eating freely has now been reduced. Reduced bulk in the intestine can make it difficult to evacuate as you previously did. There are solutions. One is to drink plenty of water. Also, use fibre supplements such as Isabgol. One to two teaspoons Isabgol in a big glass of water once or twice a day could do the trick. If constipation persists or worsens, seek medical help to relieve it with medication. A related point to make: one popular myth is to take laxatives to lose weight. Your excess weight is due to the storage of fat. It is not due to accumulation of faecal matter. The laxatives could get rid of faecal matter and temporarily show a slight reduction in weight (about half-a-kg at the most). However, laxatives have no effect on the stored fat. Moreover, abuse of some strong laxatives may even hurt your health.

How quickly does the weight drop?

It is biology. Not math: A few years ago, a theory was promoted that if you eat twenty fewer calories a day, it will translate to 365 x 20 = 7,300 calories less per year, which would mean a loss of about 1 kg per year. Ten kg loss in 10 years, by reducing just 20 calories in a day – equivalent to 1 teaspoon of sugar. Of course this attractive mathematical calculation is very convenient to promote the view that achieving weight loss is this simple. Unfortunately, it does not apply to real life human biology for many reasons. First of all, it is almost impossible to accurately achieve and determine a reduction of 20 calories in the entire day. There are too many other factors such as all the other food we may eat or avoid, or the activity for the day that may vary, which determine if we are in calorie surplus or deficit by the end of a day. Simply put, a mathematical calculation of weight loss based on daily calorie deficit does not work in real life. Why am I sharing this sombre news with you? So that you can have the right expectations from your weight loss programme. If you are now eating about 500 calories less than your daily requirement, don't let the Internet convince you that you will be losing 2 kg per month, 24 kg in a year and 48 kg in two years. This is not what happens in reality. For best results, you do have to follow the diet accurately. However, even after following the diet, your weight loss cannot be accurately predicted. This point cannot be overemphasized. We humans are naturally inclined to comparing our weight loss to that of others and we often find some examples that make us feel disheartened because of those who have lost weight much faster. *Stop comparing your weight loss.* Your response is going to be unique to your circumstances. Focus just on your progress.

You lose more weight in early days: During the early days of a diet, weight loss is very rapid. Do not calculate your weight loss journey based on the first week's loss. Two kg in first week will not translate to 8 kg per month for the next six months. This is because the initial weight loss is mainly due to the loss of water accumulated, but little loss of fat. Once you lose the initial water, you will continue to lose some water later, but it will not be as dramatic. This amount is highly variable among individuals. It is generally proportional to your initial weight. If you are above 100 kg, in the first week, you may experience even 2 to 3 kg water loss. If you are closer to 70 kg, the water loss may be 1–2 kg. However, if you have already been on a different weight loss diet or have been off and on dieting, you are not likely to see as dramatic a water loss in the initial weeks. This is important to note because the initial rapid weight loss may get you unduly enthused and raise expectations, only to disappoint you later if the loss in weight in the second or third week is less impressive. Many individuals unnecessarily quit dieting during this period because they do not understand or anticipate this natural phenomenon.

Weight decrease is not a straight line down: As the weight loss progresses, the proportion of water lost will reduce and the proportion of fat loss will increase, along with some loss in muscle. But the weight loss will not occur in a continuous straight line. Instead, it will be in a stepladder manner. You may lose weight daily for a day or two and then there may be no weight loss for three or four days, followed by another sudden drop in weight, and so on. At times, you may not lose for a week, and then see a sudden drop. This is another landmine for a dieter, who could get frustrated to not see a change in weight despite best efforts and may simply give up. Therefore, it is best to not weigh obsessively every day, but perhaps once in a week or two. Daily weighing is also not advised because body water content changes daily and between morning and evening. Therefore, unless there is substantial loss in weight, the readings could be misleading. Measuring fat loss instead of just weight loss is a much better approach to track your success.

What to do if weight loss stops?

It is inevitable that sometime despite dieting, weight loss will stop. You may lose, say, 10 kg and things just seem to come to a grinding halt. You used to lose a kg a week and now even when you are trying the same, you have barely lost half-a-kg in the past three weeks. What happened? Many people hit this phase about four months into dieting, whereas some others encounter it after six to eight months. Very few continue a smooth ride to their goal without interruption. Also, you are likely to face this situation more than once. Here is how to respond when your weight loss slows down or stops unexpectedly. Except when you hit the last step of plateau described below, it is most likely that weight loss will resume as you address each possibility described below.

- **Are you losing fat?**: It is possible that you are in fact losing fat, but not able to notice due to some water retention. This can easily be determined by focusing on fat loss instead of weight loss, by using the body composition scale that shows body weight as well as body fat content. Compare the amount of fat you had three weeks ago to what it is now. Is there a difference? Another approach is to rely on the measurements of waist and hips circumference. If you continue to lose fat, your scale will indicate so, and you will have also lost inches of your waist or hips. In that case, you continue the diet and the fat loss will continue and weight will eventually show a reduction. If there is no fat loss for three weeks, it is time to go to the next step of examining your adherence to diet.

- **Double-check if you are really following the diet**: The next question is to examine closely and candidly if you are really following the diet. Often, we are very enthusiastic and careful about the diet initially. After some weight loss, and a few months into it, some of us start taking success for granted. You also get tired of restricting diet and controlling temptations. You start taking some liberties with the diet here and there. Previously, you were very rigid even when you ate out or attended parties. Now, your friends or relatives praise your weight loss, and pressure you a bit and you start giving in. Unfortunately, this is also the time when body's calorie requirement is reducing because of your weight loss. So, at a time when you should be stricter and more disciplined about your diet, your grip on the diet starts slipping. It is also only human to slack off a bit after weeks or months of strict dieting. Perfectly understandable. But, unfortunately, you cannot have it both ways. It is only natural that you will not get returns in terms of weight loss, if your efforts have reduced. If you are going to cheat occasionally, then do not expect the same rate of weight loss. It would be a willing and intentional compromise.

- **Tighten your belt**: Eventually, weight loss can stop no matter how fully you are committed to and compliant with the diet. You are not deviating from diet and continuing as always and yet the weight has come to a standstill. It could be frustrating when this happens. You are trying everything possible, have very carefully examined your adherence to diet and yet see that weight loss has stopped. No need to panic. This is just an indication that it is time to reduce the number of calories you are eating, or increase activity further. This is the reason one weight-loss diet does not last forever and you need to further reduce caloric intake. In the chapter on diets (chapter 4, Table 5), simply go to the next lower level calories of diet and you should see weight loss again.

Just this summer, a dietitian called me for advice about a middle-aged patient who had started on a weight loss diet. The patient lost 12 kg in the first ten weeks. Thereafter, the weight did not move for two months, no matter how hard she tried and how strictly the patient followed the diet. After discussing the case, it was clear to me that after losing 12 kg, the patient's requirement of calories had dropped and the original low-calorie diet did not pack enough punch to do the job anymore. By now, the patient was on a 1,000-calories-a-day diet. I personally do not prefer diets that provide less than 1,000 calories. Therefore, I was not willing to recommend further reduction in calories. It could also adversely affect patient's quality of life. Instead, I focused on activity. There was scope to increase her activity. She was walking about 5,000 steps a day. She could not add a lot more walking due to some knee pain. However, she fortunately had the ability and willingness to walk in a swimming pool, which reduces stress on your knees. She added 8,000 more steps per day in a pool in two sessions. That would burn up about 400 extra calories. When I heard last, she had started losing again and had lost 3 kg in the next three months. The bottom line is to remember that as you keep losing weight, the diet needs to decrease and activity needs to increase in order to keep losing weight.

- **The dreaded – but normal – plateau:** Your weight loss may stop and start through above-mentioned three phases. If you have a lot of weight to lose, eventually you will come to a point which is ill-understood but well known in scientific circles as a 'plateau'. This is a stage when your body will simply refuse to shed further weight, no matter what. This inevitable stage will come in six months to some or in two years to others. Based on what science thinks about the contributors to a weight-loss plateau, it seems possible to prolong the time when you will reach a plateau by preserving muscle mass during weight loss. This is achieved by increasing physical activity and substantial amount of high quality protein intake, as described in previous chapters. Nonetheless, it is prudent to recognize the plateau as the limit of weight loss and accept this phenomenon. At this point, it would be helpful to focus on weight maintenance instead of weight loss as described in a subsequent chapter.

Life after substantial weight loss:

After you have been dieting for some time and lost weight, your life begins to change in so many ways. Over the years, my patients have shared positive as well as negative encounters during their life after weight loss. Perhaps the most common response you will get from those seeing you for the first time after noticeable weight loss is a concern for your health. 'You lost so much weight. What's wrong with you? Were you ill?' You respond: 'Nothing wrong. Just reduced some weight.' From here, the conversation can go in one of the two directions. A small fraction of individuals will respond in a way you were hoping – to compliment you on your newly acquired health and looks, and your determination in accomplishing a difficult goal. A larger number will immediately chide you for the 'terribly thin' look you have acquired and that 'you have lost lustre from your face and skin'. Their advice will be to at once stop your diet fad. Unless borne out of jealousy, the comments are well-meaning and out of concern for you. Nonetheless, they have a big impact on those who receive them. After all, you have put in a lot of hard work for a long time. And, even though your intention was to improve health by losing weight, you will admit there is also some desire to receive compliments from your friends and relatives. You start doubting yourself when bombarded with such reactions. This self-doubt can lead to loosening of your grip on weight-loss programme. Therefore, I would like to analyse the situation to forewarn and prepare you to face it effectively.

In India, excess weight is traditionally linked to prosperity because undernourishment is linked with poverty and disease. Moreover, losing weight voluntarily is neither easy nor commonplace. Hence, when you see that someone has lost weight, it seems natural to conclude that it is due to an illness. There is also some truth to the comment about following diet fads and hurting yourself in the process. There are more so-called nutritionists who do not know nutritional science than those who will advise accurately. So, your chances of unwittingly running into a quack are much more than dieting in a scientific manner. Little wonder your near and dear ones are concerned for you. To put their mind at ease, it would be up to you to explain the scientific rigour behind your weight loss effort. It will also help to let them know that your achievement is the result of a strategic rearrangement of the regular day-to-day food, and without any pills, herbs or injections.

And, yes. About the lustre of your skin. Fat is stored under our skin, which makes the skin stretch. A stretched skin looks lighter in colour, much the same as a dark red balloon when inflated will start looking pink. This phenomenon is routinely observed during pregnancy. A stretched abdomen due to pregnancy looks much lighter in colour. When you lose fat from underneath the skin, it will look a bit darker for a brief period. You may also feel a bit of surplus skin. One of my patients lost 60 kg to come down from 130 kg to 70 kg. She was not a tall person. So, losing almost half her body weight was a very big deal. By the time she completed this amazing transformation, she was nearing seventy years of age. Due to her late age and weight loss, she experienced extra skinfolds especially around her arms and abdomen. She consulted a plastic surgeon, who helped get rid of the extra skin. Unless the weight loss amount is too huge, this measure is not needed for most, whose skin simply adjusts to the new body shape.

Summary

It is not enough to know how to drive a car, but it is also important to be familiar with driving rules and regulations of the country or place you will be driving in. Much the same way, it is not enough to start a weight-loss diet without first learning what to expect next and how to navigate through it. Just like driving safely is not only about your driving, but also in response to other cars and pedestrians around, your weight loss does not happen in isolation, but in the society that you live in. Therefore, you need to be prepared to respond to their reactions as well. Following are some key points to note as you embark on the weight-loss journey.

Early changes

Improvement in energy levels; feeling energetic.

Reductions in elevated insulin, glucose or blood pressure even before substantial weight loss. Remember to adjust the dose if taking medications to lower these conditions.

Improvement in feeling of heaviness or bloating. If it persists, check with doctor for other causes.

Constipation. Address by increasing water and fibre intake.

As weight loss starts

Not possible to predict how much or how fast you will lose. It varies.

Weight loss is faster initially. This is mainly due to rapid loss of water.

Weight loss is not a straight line down. It starts and stops and proceeds in a stepladder manner.

When weight loss stops

Check if fat loss is still continuing

Tighten your grip on following the diet, if slipping

Reduce the calorie intake to next lower level or increase activity

Face and accept the plateau.

After noticeable weight loss

Expect well-meaning comments from friends and family. Explain your scientific approach to weight loss and health gain.

8

Sorry! I'm on a Diet

During the three weeks he stayed at a U.S. resort, Mr Aamir Khan lost 6 kg. The reason we decided to take this step in his weight loss was to take him away from society and to be in an environment that did not present social challenges. With no social occasions, no festivals, no business lunches and no travel, there would be no temptations. Just the diet and exercise plan. Period. Indeed, if we all didn't live in a society, we too may lose way more weight. But that's not realistic. It's smart to recognize the rules of the games and plan accordingly.

I have seen people complain about India having too many festivals and food-centred celebrations and hospitality that interfere with their weight loss. So? Are you waiting for a time when no one celebrates festivals? Will you never attend another wedding, or party, or go to eat at a restaurant? That sounds like quite an unpleasant life by usual standards. Instead, it's better to devise a plan that helps you navigate these diet landmines, so that you can live in this society and yet improve your health.

Selecting a good diet and exercise plan is a must for good weight loss and health improvement. But, a good 'plan' is not enough. We need effective and skilful execution of this plan. One still has to deal with external as well as internal pressures that frustrate dieters. Let's face those pressures head on and devise some key strategies that can save a diet plan in peril.

Generally, external pressures come from well-meaning friends and family. India has a history of famine. Therefore, overweight is traditionally considered a positive sign of health and prosperity. During the times when food abundance was not common and undernutrition prevailed, the only safeguard against bad effects of diseases, like tuberculosis, was keeping the bodyweight high by eating plenty of food. Indeed, in 1800s, if you ate 'well' and had plenty of reserve energy, you were likely to survive many infectious diseases that were prevalent at the time. Hence, our cultures, festivities, hosts, relatives, even spouses, seek to feed us. Understanding this underlying reason will help you see the good intentions of those who are lovingly asking you to eat more. The problem is, that in this time of plenty, your body does not need that excess food during your weight-loss plan, and your loved ones' hospitality weakens your re-solve.

That brings us to internal pressures, within you, which also weigh heavily on a dieter's mind. Wanting to eat food is a natural and normal desire – third most important survival need of the body, after air and water. Our mind is subconsciously looking for an opportunity to eat, and disregard any dietary restrictions. Temptations are inevitable and normal to humans. There are multiple strategies to steer clear of such temptations, and make it easier to fight the internal pressures that push us towards eating excess calories. Let's examine these possibilities. A couple of disclosures: 1) Some of these strategies are a result of my clinical experience and they have worked for umpteen number of my patients, but they are not necessarily borrowed from published research in the field. In that sense, these strategies are unique and original 2) Not all strategies apply to each person. Follow the ones that best suit your specific circumstances.

1. **Sorry. I am on a diet**: In an earlier chapter, we discussed recruiting the help of friends and family before embarking on a diet plan. But that may not cover all your acquaintances. You will certainly be in situations when you must make a choice between respecting host's feelings or protecting your health. While each situation may be different, my recommendation is to get that host on your side. It is hard to keep your dieting a secret. You are most likely to appear rude, and unappreciative of the food made if you just eat little, without any explanation. Instead, candidly admit to the host that you are following a diet plan, state that it is for your health, and ask the host for their help in assisting you to stick to your plan. The earlier you do this in the interaction, the better it is. If you know about the party or dinner beforehand,

it is better to let the host know about your diet days in advance, than springing a surprise upon them at the last moment. Having various food restrictions is not at all unusual for an Indian household. Remember, how many people observe different dietary restrictions for religious fasts? Some don't eat non-vegetarian on Tuesdays, no eggs during a month, or eat only white-coloured food on Fridays and so on. We convey these religion-based food restrictions to hosts regularly and these are honoured and accommodated easily by the hosts. No questions asked. Try the exact same route for your weight-loss diet.

2. **Illusion**: While making no secret about your weight-loss diet is a good idea, it is probably impractical to announce about your diet during big events such as a large office party or a wedding reception. And you don't have to. The hosts are probably too busy looking after too many other guests. In these situations, you just have to avoid the *appearance* of eating less. Now, it is true that we grow up hearing, 'Food should not be left on the plate. Clean your plate. Eat everything.' The point of this admonishment is that food should not be wasted, and you should be served only the amount that you will not waste. I agree. However, given the option, I would rather waste that food in my plate than overeat and allow it to remain on my waist. During certain events, people around you will immediately notice if you start dinner with little food on the plate. This will be followed by every comment to

sabotage your diet. Instead, a time-tested approach is to fill your plate normally, just like how others are doing, but then eat only what you wish. Then there is no cause for alarm for your friends and no one will follow you around to see how much of the food remained on your plate when you discarded it. Believe me, it works.

3. **BYOF**: Bring Your Own Food. I knew a district governor of Rotary International, who during his term as governor, had to attend hundreds of events. This meant facing hundreds of tempting meals in presence of very hospitable and caring fellow Rotarians. Normally, maintaining a diet or healthy weight would have been out of the question for him. So, his solution was to carry his own 'tiffin' everywhere, so he could attend those events and yet maintain health as well. After the initial surprise, people around him grew accustomed to this quirk and nobody bothered him about it. Many a times, the inhibitions you feel are mainly in your mind. At times, it helps to expose others to somewhat unconventional approaches and inform them about your priorities. You can politely send a message that interactions, networking, friendly chat or other business do not always have to depend on food and at times, you would participate in all that and enjoy, but will BYOF.

4. **Dinner before dinner**: This is a combination of principles of strategies 1, 2 and 3 above, see if this suits you better. For this approach, you eat dinner at home before going

for a social dinner. When you arrive, let the host know politely that you are on a diet and that you would really appreciate if you are not forced too much to eat, that you would like to enjoy the food but within limits. After this explanation to your hosts and others, and with a full stomach (because you have had the dinner earlier), you may then eat that paneer kabab or chicken tikka or have only half a piece of naan with very little navratan korma. The critical point is that in such situation, you will eat only for the taste and not to fill your stomach (since you have already eaten at home). That makes a big difference on the food quantity eaten and in calories consumed. This approach simultaneously accommodates your own temptations, shows respect to the hosts and their efforts and gives you a way to limit calories. Hunger is our worst enemy when it comes to controlling temptations.

It will probably occur to you that I am advocating against a popular practice of 'starving' the whole day in anticipation of a heavy meal at night. You reason that 'I will be eating a lot of calories at night. Might as well save some calories by eating less during the day.' But that is not likely to work. Here's why. In the USA, it is routinely recommended to not go weekly grocery shopping on an empty stomach. You will be surprised about the number and type of foods purchased when you are full versus when starving. You will be tempted to buy a lot more food if hungry. And, of course, foods that come home from the stores, usually ends up in you. The same logic applies here. Imagine attending a wedding reception with stalls for bhel puri, pani-puri, chaat, and Mexican, Italian or Indian foods, and mouth-watering starters and desserts. Now, you can predict the outcome if you attend this feast on an empty stomach versus on a full stomach. I bet you are getting thoughts about food just reading this – especially if you are hungry.

Which Diet Personality Type are You?

Not everything about successful dieting is about dealing with others. There are also some internal factors, some struggles or behaviours to recognize and to overcome within ourselves. These are your dietary personalities. I should mention politely yet matter-of-factly, that a major reason why my patients have enjoyed high success with weight loss is because of the effort I invest in understanding their dietary personality type and counselling them accordingly. I know too well that one shoe size does not fit all. One diet and one diet approach is not suitable for all. So, here I am sharing my strategies for your benefit. See which ones apply to you.

a. **The Grazers:** I, personally, am a Grazer. As kids, we would visit my mother's parents' home during summer vacations. Food would be truly plentiful, but was offered three times a day. Breakfast, lunch and dinner. Snacks between meals were not common. If hungry at odd times, we were asked to drink milk. My personal preference on the other hand is to eat small and frequent meals. Overall, I get full easily and feel hungry soon. As a kid, I would find myself going through the kitchen in between meals.

Eating three big square meals is not my style. So, now I eat a small breakfast at 7 a.m. (typically half a bagel, equivalent to say about a bread slice), a small snack at 10:00 a.m., then lunch at 12 noon, followed by snacks at 3:00 p.m., dinner at 8 p.m. and again something before bedtime. These snacks are not elaborate meals and are quick enough to suit my work style of constant meetings, phone calls and conversations. Some examples of such snacks would be 10 cherries or 15 almonds or half a protein bar or a small bottle of Frappuccino coffee. If you are a grazer, try dividing your food in many small meals. If you are not, there's no need to eat frequent meals. In fact, you may end up eating much more if that is not your style. Stick to the number of meals that you are comfortable with. No need to take on someone else's diet personality.

b. Firm or flexible: Some individuals prefer consistency in their diet pattern. For them, it is easy to stick to one dietary pattern and it is easier if there are not too many choices in the diet. That is the **Firm** dietary personality. Variation is neither needed nor tolerated by these personalities. On the other hand, the **Flexible** personalities have a hard time sticking to one type of dietary behaviour. They require some variation, some change from daily diet. Perhaps, a change in diet pattern on a weekend. They are not necessarily seeking to stop dieting over the weekend, but just a little respite in the routine. The Firm personality cannot handle this variation. If they make a small variation, they seem to lose the grip on their programme. It is hard for them to get back to the routine. Just think and figure out where you stand. No need to blindly follow what works for your friends. What works for you is important.

c. **All or nothing**: It is normal to be tempted by some calorie-rich foods that you have been avoiding during a weight-loss diet. Let's say, chocolate or ice cream is your weakness, which you miss the most when on a diet. There are two approaches to deal with this, depending on your diet personality. It is possible that curbing such temptations completely for a long time could make some feel miserable and may reduce the overall quality of life. It will not be good if this frustration leads to just quitting the programme entirely. Instead, a strategy is needed to respond to those temptations. Say, if you find yourself day-dreaming about ice cream, it is much better to just go ahead and eat some. The key word here is 'some'. It is the amount that matters. Eat some and stop. Is it even possible and is it realistic? Indeed possible, if you follow exactly as I describe: First, do not satisfy these food cravings on an empty stomach. The point is to not eat these calorie-rich foods to fill your stomach, but only for the taste of it. Rule 2: Do not eat directly from a container or package. Scoop out that ice cream from its container in a bowl for your use, or break off the pieces of chocolate you need from the slab, or take out a piece of that ras malai in your bowl. Now, start eating and notice that after initial few bites, you are likely to have satisfied the craving. If so, stop. No need to finish everything that you served yourself. Most people can stop eating and limit the intake, once they satisfy their initial craving. Even if you did not follow the diet strictly, this approach helps preserve the quality of life.

On the other hand, some individuals may need a very different strategy. I had a patient who absolutely loved jalebi, the fried and sugar syrup infused delicious bomb of calories. She ate them every day. When I was planning her diet, and contemplating about how to accommodate jalebis at least once a week or so, her response was very telling of this type of personality. She categorically mentioned that she ate ½ kg jalebi daily, and could eat more. Eating one occasionally was not going to work for her. The only way to not eat ½ kg jalebi was to not eat it at all. There was no middle ground, no compromise when it came to this. It was much easier for her to be not exposed to the temptations at all than to have to limit the number. I have seen this approach in many individuals who wish to totally abstain from their problem foods, instead of tasting a little bit. This is the **All or Nothing** personality. You know how you respond. Choose your approach accordingly.

A note about sweets and desserts, which have a very bad reputation in the world of dieting and weight loss. Because of their sweet taste, people consider sugar as evil and high in calories. In fact, sugar and protein have the same number of calories, 4 per gram. It is the fat content of that dessert which makes all the difference in terms of calories. Fat has 9 calories per gram. So, jalebis are not high in calories because of sugar, but because they are deep fried and have a lot of fat. In an ice cream, about half the calories come from the fat. The point is to be careful about foods that have high fat and not worry as much about foods that taste sweet. In Indian desserts, the sweet taste is guilty only by its association with fat. For example, jelly or jam taste very sweet, but have no fat. So, they are not calorie-rich. If you must eat something to satisfy your sweet tooth, hard candy, jelly, jam, syrup are relatively lower calorie options.

d. **Delayed fullness:** The 'hunger hormones' in the body signal to us when we are hungry, which helps start a meal. As we eat, a set of 'fullness hormones' rise in the blood and signal satiety, so we can stop eating. The response of these hunger or satiety hormones varies in different individuals, which may explain why some of us take much longer to feel full when eating a meal. This delayed feeling of fullness could make you eat more food. For every minute delay in the onset of satiety, you could be eating 70 calories extra. So, if your feeling of fullness is delayed by 5 minutes compared someone else's, you may eat about 350 extra calories during that period. It is not a good situation when trying to lose weight. However, if that is simply how your body functions, there are ways around it. It is a simple approach and we already discussed it earlier. Drink water.

Drink a glass of water towards the end of your meal, say when you are about three-fourth done. A sudden fullness will kick in, allowing you to easily make the right decision of terminating the meal earlier and saving you from taking in extra calories. This is no rocket science, yet a very effective trick of inducing fullness earlier. Note that it does not help much if you drank that same amount of water before starting the meal.

e. **Eating disorders:** It is important to talk about two key disorders while discussing diet personalities. They are Bulimia Nervosa and Binge Eating Disorder.

Bulimia involves eating a large amount of food in an uncontrolled manner, followed by a huge feeling of guilt, which drives a person to repent and undertake some seemingly corrective measure such as inducing vomiting to throw up that food or to take laxatives to pass stools. Inducing vomiting repeatedly and chronically is harmful to health. Laxative abuse is not good and passing stools does not correct what you already ate.

A person with the Binge Eating Disorder also indulges in a binge, but without the vomiting behaviour or laxative use.

A binge is not just a bit of overeating, but a truly enormous amount of food. As an example, a binge could include a full big pack of ice cream, 4 slabs of chocolates, 2 big bags of potato chips, two bowls of cereal, 3 plates of bhel and so on, all eaten in one sitting within a small timespan. If any of these two fits the description of behaviour for you or your friends or family, an expert's advice is the best option. This is less of a nutritional issue and more psychological. It should be addressed by a psychologist or psychiatrist trained to handle these conditions. To impress upon your mind the need to seek professional mental health in these situations, I will not even discuss the treatment options here. Please see an expert.

SUMMARY

Selecting a good diet and exercise plan is a must for good weight loss and health improvement. However, having a good plan is not enough. Its effective and skilful execution is also needed. In a world full of temptations and well-meaning friends and family, who inadvertently test your diet resolve, two main strategies to maximize the weight loss benefits are as follows

1. **Learn to pre-empt high-risk situations**
   a. **Sorry. I am on a diet:** Candidly declare that you are on a diet, and seek your host's help in sticking to the diet.

b. **Illusion:** In a big party or event, you may be teased about the diet, if you start the meal with little food. Instead, no one notices if you start with normal amount, but eat only as much you want.

c. **BYOF:** If you really mean business, simply carry your food to an event or a party. People may be surprised initially, but then get over it.

d. **Dinner before dinner:** Have dinner at home before attending a party. Because you are not hungry, at the party you will only eat little of that calorie-rich food, just for the taste of it.

2. **Recognize your diet personality:**

a. **The grazers:** You may need to divide the daily food quota in many small meals.

b. **Firm or flexible**: Either you cannot handle variation, or need some change in diet routine from time to time. Do what suits you best.

c. **All or nothing:** It may satisfy you to try only a little bite of highly tempting food, instead of totally avoiding it. This may help preserve the quality of life. Alternatively, you may be of the type that once you start eating something, you are unable to control yourself. In that case, it is better to not be exposed to tempting foods while on a diet.

d. **Delayed fullness:** In some, feeling full after a meal takes some time, which may substantially increase the calories eaten during a meal. Drinking a glass of water towards the end of a meal does the magic of hastening satiety.

e. **Eating disorders:** If you have any of these eating disorders, do not fight them alone. Get expert advice and care.

9

Maintaining Fat Loss

I should have mentioned earlier that before he started obesity practice in 1962, my father's first patient was he himself. He experimented on himself to lose weight from 100 kg to 64 kg. What was most impressive was that he remained within a couple of kg of that weight throughout his life. This was a remarkable achievement in weight maintenance, which he also taught to his patients, and to me. It did not come without a price. I saw him practise the art of good nutrition and activity all my life. For him, the alternative of weight regain was not pleasant. Those of you have experienced weight regain know how frustrating it is. It is not easy to prevent regain, but it certainly is possible.

Weight maintenance is needed to obtain long-term health benefits. Think of diabetes. It is not enough to reduce the blood sugar to normal level if you are not going to maintain it. Same is true with body fat or body weight. Even if you are vigilant, weight maintenance is not guaranteed. You experienced weight gain in the first place because you have the tendency to gain weight. That tendency remains even after you lose weight. I agree that it is not fair that you have to watch weight all your life, while some other lucky people never ever worry about theirs. Unfair indeed; but that's how things are. So, instead of griping about the unfairness of it all, let's learn the rules of the game and then play it masterfully.

Many of my patients have successfully maintained weight loss. Their individual strategies for weight maintenance may differ slightly. However, some commonalities among those who were successful stand out. These individuals typically have the burning concern to maintain weight and health and a desire to be vigilant and to not let go. They are ready to pay the price in terms of efforts needed to maintain. They consider weight loss as 'phase one' and weight maintenance as 'phase two' – two very distinct phases. They do not declare victory after the first phase. Their outlook is more long-term than settling for a quick fix. In general, I observed that these individuals were not perturbed by some minor setbacks, but kept in mind the larger perspective of health that lasts a lifetime. Here is an outline of the nine rules that I recommended for long-term and effective weight maintenance. Each rule is important, but they produce best results when followed together.

1. **Keep track**: The absolute top priority is to keep track of your body weight. Whether dieting or not, weigh yourself regularly and note it down. If you find yourself forgetting to weigh and note down, I can bet you will not maintain weight. Only if you're serious about losing weight will

you regularly keep track of it. Daily weight will fluctuate, sometimes, even by 1.5 kg. However, your weight records will make it easy to differentiate between fluctuations and an upward trend over time.

2. **Hydrate**: Water continues to be important in weight loss and weight maintenance. Your aim should be drinking about two litres of water in a day. It is okay to carry a bottle of water with you. People will get used to seeing you with a bottle and you will get used to sipping water throughout the day. This will help you reduce temptations and keep you from feeling exhausted, in addition to the good effects of water on daily metabolism. I'm often asked whether tea or coffee could be counted in two litres of water. The answer is yes. However, it is better if you drink two litres of water in addition to other sources of fluid.

3. **Step up:** Many scientific studies have shown that physical activity is even more important for weight maintenance than during weight loss. If you have lost weight as per the suggestions in the previous chapters, by now you must be used to walking for exercise. If you were walking about 10,000 steps a day for weight loss, try to increase it to 12,000 to 15,000 steps a day during weight maintenance. Of course, walking is not the only type of physical activity or exercise and the benefits of exercise depend on the kind of exercise. Now that you have lost weight, you may want to add that sport or game you have always wanted to play, but could not when you were heavier. Or you

could undertake muscle building, toning or training for developing cardiovascular endurance. It is a good idea to consult a physical trainer in determining your workout routine and guard against any injuries arising from wrong workouts.

4. **Increase calories:** You will not be on a weight *loss* diet to maintain weight. You can actually eat more than what you were eating to lose weight, and yet maintain. As mentioned in the previous chapters, to lose weight, you have to first determine the total calories you need for a day and then eat fewer calories than your requirement. For example, if you needed 2,200 calories for a day and you chose a diet of 1,800 calories, you were eating 400 calories fewer a day to lose weight. Now, for weight maintenance, you needn't continue eating less. Recalculate the number of calories you will need at your new weight. Remember that your body weight is a big determinant of the caloric need. So, after weight loss, plug in your new weight in the formula and obtain the calories you need now. If they were 2,200 initially, after weight loss the new need may be, say, 1,950. So, you will be able to increase calories from 1,800 from your weight loss days to 1,950 and still be able to maintain weight. This is a very important concept. The key, however, is to not overeat. You still must be vigilant and careful in selecting what and how much you eat. That vigilance is needed as long as you wish to maintain weight.

5. **Follow the diet principles**: When maintaining weight, follow the same general diet principles of a weight-loss diet. Remember the Protein Shield? Protein-containing foods such as eggs, fish, chicken, meat, pulses, beans, legumes, lentils and daals, offer significant protection from hunger, which you need during the day. Therefore, during weight maintenance, it continues to be important to include protein-rich foods in sufficient quantity during the day instead of eating them only at night, before going to bed.

    Typically, the 'weight-loss phase' is relatively shorter, compared to the 'weight-maintenance phase', which in theory, should be for the rest of your life. The main objective of the former phase is to focus on calories and reduce weight. Proper nutrition is by all means extremely important, but it is second on the priority list during that phase. During the 'weight-maintenance phase', this objective shifts. You still have to be watchful about calories. But considering that this phase will last forever, receiving complete nutrition is more important.

    Food provides us calories, carbohydrates, proteins, fats, various vitamins and minerals, and fibre, all of which are necessary for health. The focus of the weight-maintenance phase is on obtaining all these essential nutrients in required quantities while also maintaining the weight. The key to getting these nutrients through diet on a regular basis is variety. Breakfast cereals such as oats; staple foods such as rice, wheat, jowar or bajra; vegetables like root vegetables, green leafy vegetables, salads, carrots; sources of protein such as different varieties of lentils and beans, eggs, meat or fish; citrus fruits such as oranges and lemons; or mango, banana, grapes, dates; nuts such as walnut, peanuts, or almonds; milk, curds, all provide many unique nutrients. They are too numerous to list. But, for example, the basic nutrients such as milk proteins, milk sugar, calcium, etc., are similar in milk and curds. In addition, though, curds provide bacteria that are helpful to the gut. Similarly, fruits are very good for us but different fruits specialize in providing different nutrients. You eat an orange to get a strong dose of vitamin C, whereas a mango provides a lot of vitamin A. You have heard that salads are good for us. Again, the ingredients matter. Carrots would be a great source of vitamin A, whereas, spinach or other dark green leafy vegetables would be higher in iron content. You get the idea. Each food has something special to offer for our health. *Hence, variation is the key.*

If you are a rice eater, include occasional chapattis or rotis of wheat flour, or even some of jowar or bajra. Mix and match foods frequently and you may not need to take nutrient supplements. Another rule of thumb some researchers recommend is to look at the colour of food in your plate. Your plate should be as colourful as possible. It should not be only brown or yellow colour, but should have green, red, orange, yellow, pink, white and so on.

You can imagine the colours of a plate containing green vegetables, red bell peppers, melon or mango, curds, rice, dal, beans. Foods, when wisely selected, should be able to supply nutrients adequately in a normal healthy person.

6. **Fats need special attention**: The rule about variety also applies to fats in our diet, which we get from two main sources. One source is the fat present in various foods, such as coconut, peanut and other nuts, corn, meats and fish, milk and even fruits like avocado. The other source of fats is cooking oil, which is added to foods. While all these fats, regardless of their food source, provide same number of calories (9 calories per gram), their effects on health differ. While the calorie content of these fats is especially important during the weight-loss phase, the health effects have important consideration during the maintenance phase. Fats from fish, known as fish oil or omega-3 fats have many health benefits. Similarly, fats from peanuts and other nuts are considered desirable, relative to some other fats known as saturated fats, which don't have a good reputation. Saturated fats readily provide raw material to the body to make cholesterol. While cholesterol is a useful substance, in excess quantities it can get deposited in blood vessels and invite trouble such as heart disease. We obtain cholesterol directly from foods such as eggs, meat, chicken, etc., or our body can make its own cholesterol from saturated fats. Recent research shows that food sources of cholesterol such as

eggs are the leading contributors to body's cholesterol as much saturated fat. A big supplier of saturated fats is milk fat in the form of cream, ghee, butter, cheese and other sweet made from milk. In the long-term, it is important to limit the intake of saturated fats, especially if high blood cholesterol levels is a concern.

While on this topic, let me address a popular belief about weight maintenance. A recent theory proclaims that eating ghee does wonders for the body, including helping you lose and maintain weight. In fact, one of my recent patients mentioned a weight-loss diet given by another individual before she started consulting me. She was asked to eat at least ten teaspoons of ghee every day. Ten teaspoons of ghee has about 450 calories. These extra calories in ghee were supposed to help her lose weight. Instead, during that year-long treatment, she gained 10 kg. Needless to say, she discontinued this extra intake of calories when I prescribed a diet.

This theory deserves a word or two here. Twenty-five years ago, when I was a researcher at the University of Wisconsin in Madison, Wisconsin, I worked closely with Professor Michael Pariza, the famous researcher credited for promoting conjugated linoleic acid, or CLA, as a possible treatment against weight gain. CLA is found in substantial amount in ghee and at the time, my Indian mind recognized the opportunity to brag about the ancient wisdom about using ghee for weight loss. Many experiments in animals successfully showed that CLA reduced weight gain. My hopes were gaining strength. However, subsequent studies done in humans produced weak results, if any. While CLA research for different health benefits continues, the hope of using CLA for weight loss have all but vanished. Although it has been several years since we know that CLA or CLA-containing ghee is not going to be a magic bullet for weight loss, perhaps the news is slow in travelling to India, where it is a popular prescription by some 'weight-loss experts'. In addition, ghee has the same number of calories as in other oils. Moreover, ghee has saturated fats, the ones that the body uses for making cholesterol. None of these provides a good reason for increasing ghee intake during weight loss or maintenance. Although it sounds attractive and evokes patriotic emotions about an indigenous food like ghee, it will not help you. Also, it is medically untrue that that ghee lubricates knee joints and other joints. Our joints are lubricated by synovial fluid, which is comprised of complex chemicals made from glucose and proteins. Eating ghee does not find its way directly into the joints.

7. **Beware of the hidden calories**: During the weight-loss phase, your food choices were limited. You were required to eat specific food types in specified quantities. During the weight maintenance phase, you are likely to be exposed to everything that is available. Therefore, an awareness of calorie content of food is critical during this phase.

One plate of two samosas can give as many as 800 to 900 calories, which is roughly equivalent to 14 slices of bread, and you may need to walk up to 15 km to burn off just those calories. This example highlights the issue of hidden calories in foods. The very high calorie value of samosas is not due to the wheat pastry cover or the potato stuffing, but the oil that was used for frying it. Yet, our mind never sees the oil. To make matters worse, oil is literally invisible. So, we count food as two rotis, a bowl of vegetables and dal, two fruits, etc., without ever mentioning the oil needed to cook that food. These hidden calories can sabotage your weight maintenance plan even when you seem to be eating a reasonable amount of food. In fact, it is the richness of the food, known as calorie density (calories per gram of food), and not the quantity, that matters. You could eat large amounts of food like watermelon, which has low calorie density, but you will have to limit the intake of a cake or ras malai, which are very calorie dense foods. Another example of the need for looking out for hidden calories. Puffed rice (kurmura / mamra) was included in the diet as snacks of one of my patients from the state of Maharashtra. He informed me that as advised, he was eating an equivalent snack of spiced puffed rice which is called bhadang, from the Kolhapur area of Maharashtra. It turns out that bhadang is not quite the calorie equivalent of puffed rice. Preparation of bhadang can include peanuts, some coconut and oil. Therefore, the calories in 100 g puffed rice will be about 360, but up to 900 in 100 g bhadang. These are the hidden calories, in fried or oily foods, that you need to watch out for, as you start weight maintenance.

8. **Have your cake and eat it too**: Undoubtedly, it is the oil, butter, or ghee that makes food taste great. Frying makes food crispy and tasty and oil makes butter chicken or paneer makhani delicious. Less oil means less taste. But, more oil also means more calories. What then is a practical and realistic alternative to not eating any good-tasting food and living like a hermit? Here are some tips to enjoy some yummy foods as well as to reduce the hidden calories from those foods.

   a. Reduce oil use: Use a cooking oil spray to coat the pan, instead of pouring oil from the bottle in the pan for cooking.

   b. Replace oil, when possible: For preparing foods like aloo tikki or potato patties, spray with oil and grill in the oven. Agreed that it will not taste exactly like the fried version, but the huge calorie saving may be worth it.

   c. Shallow fry, if you must: Use shallow frying, instead of deep frying.

   d. If fried, drain oil: If you fry say, bhajiya, place them in a tilted plate on a paper that would soak oil. You will be amazed to see how much oil can be drained without compromising on the good taste.

e. Pick food from oil: If you have ordered chicken masala in a restaurant, and if you are watching calories, you are likely to eat little, if any, of the piece of chicken and instead eat the gravy. You should do the opposite. It is the gravy that has all the oil. Eat less of the gravy and you will save on calories.

f. Reduce unnecessary sugar: Make it a point to not drink sugar-sweetened beverages. Those provide a lot of sugar calories in a glass of water. Instead, if you wish to drink colas, their diet counterparts are freely available and these have zero calories. And yes, they are safe to drink and not poisonous.

g. Reduce food without missing it: Burgers or sandwiches generally have one bread buttered or with mayonnaise. Remove that bread. You will eat fewer calories and yet enjoy the sandwich or the burger. Skin of chicken contains a lot of fat. Make tandoori chicken without the skin. Worth the calorie savings.

h. Dilute calories: At times, people enjoy roasted peanuts as a snack. Peanuts have about 600 calories per 100 g (equivalent of about eight slices of bread) and can quickly add calories. Whereas, roasted grams (channa) has less than 350 calories per 100 g. By mixing channa with peanuts, you can dilute the calories from peanuts. Mixing ice cream with fruits is another example of diluting high calories of ice cream with lower calories from fruits.

i. Substitution: If the preparation is the same, a fish dish will have fewer calories than chicken and a chicken dish is preferable to a mutton dish. Eggless mayonnaise has less than half the calories compared to regular mayonnaise. The same is true for a light salad dressing compared to equivalent regular dressing. In some cultures, eating root vegetables is preferred for religious fasting. Root vegetables, yam, sweet potato and potatoes rank in decreasing order of calorie content. So, choosing potatoes may be better over the other two.

9. **Follow the 3:1 rule:** It is quite possible for your weight to inch upwards even after following all the above listed suggestions. The rise could be very slow and almost imperceptible. But, your weight diary will come in handy and will let you know if your weight is really creeping up. No need to panic. This is a very common situation and completely addressable with what I refer to as the *3:1 Rule*.

Those, who cannot maintain weight with the strategies outlined above need to revisit weight loss from time to time. The time is of your choosing. You may enjoy weight maintenance for three days, followed by one day of weight loss diet. 3:1. Or, it could be three weeks of weight maintenance followed by one week of weight loss. Or, three months of weight maintenance followed by one month of weight loss. This approach allows you to enjoy a somewhat liberal weight management diet, followed by a stricter weight loss period to bring back the scale that may have crept up. Of course, the best approach is to not let the weight rise at all. However, the commitment needed for such a lifestyle may be cumbersome for many. Hence, a middle ground is to alternate between weight maintenance and weight loss at a convenient interval of your choosing.

Many ways to prevent weight gain: These are some tips to deal with weight maintenance, probably the toughest phase of weight management. Preventing weight regain is important. However, an important concept about prevention should not be overlooked. There are different categories of prevention. If you can help it, perhaps the best approach is to not let your weight go out of control in the first place (which of course is easier said than done). This is considered primary prevention. Be vigilant about the weight at all times and fight weight gain immediately even if it is as little as a kg or two, instead of waiting till the weight adds up significantly.

If you already have excess weight, the next best thing is to reduce excess weight and hold it down. That is secondary prevention. The secondary prevention may or may not be 100 per cent successful. For example, if you lose 15 kg, you may find that despite best efforts, you slowly regained 5 or 7 kg. That is still okay and better than regaining all the weight back. It may not be 100 per cent success, but there are many numbers between 0 and 100 per cent. Something is definitely better than nothing.

Finally, there is also the tertiary prevention. This means to put a stop to gaining any weight as an adult. At any weight, try to not gain weight further, even if you don't reduce it. Say you are a twenty-five-year-old woman, 5' 2" in height and weigh 75 kg. The chances are you are affected with obesity and are likely to continue to gain weight as your age advances. If you are 75 kg at twenty-five years, you may cross 85 to 90 kg by the time you reach fifty years. That is the path obesity usually takes. It is a merciless disease and if unchecked, just keeps adding the weight and weight-related health complications.

Now, imagine a situation when you fully recognize the tendency to gain weight and decide to do something about it. You fight back. With diet, exercise and other means, you try to control weight gain. After this lifelong battle, at the age of fifty or sixty, you are still 75 kg, what would be your reaction? Are you unsuccessful in the battle with obesity or successful? Sure, you did not reduce below 75 kg, but, there is a lot to be said, even if you halted the weight gain that would have almost certainly happened during your lifetime. Or, even if you changed the trajectory of weight gain and ended up gaining just a few kg in twenty-five years. These are all successes and they count. Remember that many people are struggling just like you. You are not alone. Giving up is not a good option. Arm yourself with scientific information about weight loss and maintenance such as that provided in this book. Avoid the minefield of misinformation from non-credible sources. Put in the efforts. Fight the battle. Your health is at stake. Shape it up.

Summary

Keeping the weight off is not easy, but is certainly possible. There are nine categories of suggestions for preventing weight regain.

1. **Note down**: Keep a continuous track of your weight. Forgetting to note your weight is the first step towards regaining weight.
2. **Hydrate**: Drink plenty of water. Up to 2 litres a day.
3. **Step up**: Increase your activity to 12,000 to 15,000 steps a day.
4. **Increase calories**: Unlike the weight-loss phase, during weight maintenance, you can increase the calories to match daily requirement and yet maintain weight.
5. **Follow the diet principles**: Follow the same principles of good nutrition that you used for weight loss.
6. **Fats need special attention**: Sources of fats in diet can determine if they are good or not so good fats. Not all fats are created equal. Be careful about misinformation. A lot exists.
7. **Beware of the hidden calories**: Recognize that invisible calories can do a lot of damage without you realizing it.

8. **Have your cake and eat it too**: There are ways to make slight changes in diet and foods that would preserve the quality of your life and yet help maintain weight.

9. **Follow the 3:1 rule**: Even during the weight-maintenance phase, it helps to occasionally undertake weight loss.

There are many ways to evaluate success with preventing weight gain. Each counts towards a healthy life. Don't give up.

Epilogue

Future of Obesity Management

It is sad to see so many people struggling with body weight and related health conditions. I am often inundated with pleas from people struggling to lose weight and desperate to find a solution. Researchers all over the world have made great progress in understanding this serious disease called obesity. Those of us trained to treat obesity know how to help those struggling with weight. Although not easy, it is possible to successfully lose weight and keep it off. Yet, this information does not seem to be widely available. It pains me to see many 'quacks' preying on people's helplessness. There are too many diet books in the market, which is exactly why I have written this book. I have been sitting on the sidelines for too long and have seen the rubbish theories offered by many of these books. Scientific accountability does not seem to be the concern of many who peddle baseless theories. These unscientific theories go unchallenged and soon get assimilated in society. The theories sell books, but don't help the problem. This book is my attempt to offer people a treatment that combines obesity science and my thirty-five years of experience and can help in weight loss and maintenance.

Individualized personal weight management treatment is probably most effective. However, it is not possible for me to connect with each and every individual seeking weight management. Instead, this book is an attempt to reach out to as many people possible, to spread the word about scientific approach to weight management. The book methodically covers background information about weight management and then carefully walks you through the steps of diet selection, execution and the strategies for successful weight loss and maintenance. In this sense, the book is developed to provide specific help to the extent possible. I hope that you find it useful.

This book focuses on the diet and exercise approaches to weight management. In addition, there are surgeries as well as drugs available to fight obesity. Under specific circumstances, these drugs or surgeries could be highly helpful for treating obesity for a selected population. Even when drugs or surgeries are used, diet and exercise continue to be the mainstay of obesity management. Hence, the focus of this book on diet and activity.

Drugs and surgery are also important. Like many approaches in science, obesity surgery had a bit of a rocky start. However, many of the initial surgical procedures have now been abandoned or modified such that currently popular surgical techniques have fewer adverse effects and very high success rates. Surgical approaches are mainly considered for people with high body weight, in whom the risk of excess weight outweighs the potential risk of surgery. As surgeons gain more experience and better approaches become available, surgery is becoming safer and more widely useful. Risk and success seem to depend on the technique used and the surgeon's skills. Nonetheless, it is not likely that the estimated 2.1 billion people in the world who are overweight or have obesity will receive surgery. Instead, there is a different plan envisioned.

Researchers are studying the mechanism by which obesity surgery reduces weight and improves obesity-related health conditions. For example, certain surgeries appear to improve diabetes even before substantial weight loss occurs. This surprising phenomenon is under investigation. The research is expected to reveal how the body responds to obesity surgery. It is hoped that new drugs could be developed that would mimic the action of surgery. The benefits of surgery could then be enjoyed through a pill. This, in my opinion, is the real value and gift of obesity surgery in the long run.

This brings me to the next topic that I am pinning my hopes on for obesity treatment. Obesity drugs. There are many misunderstandings regarding these. The key objections are that 1) drugs have side effects, 2) the weight comes back when you stop taking drugs and 3) why use drugs when you can lose weight with diet and exercise. Before I respond to these beliefs, note that I am referring only to legitimate drugs that are approved for obesity treatment by the Food and Drug Administration (FDA). These drugs undergo an extremely rigorous approval process by the FDA, where their beneficial and adverse effects are carefully monitored in several studies and in several thousand study participants. I am not referring to substances peddled based on hearsay benefits, without any or much official documentation. These FDA-approved obesity drugs do have side effects, like any other drugs for other conditions.

Admittedly, the earlier versions of these drugs had substantially more side effects. And, yes, they also do not work if you stop taking them. In other words, they do not work from the bottle. Why is it a surprise that you need to actually take the drugs for them to affect your body weight? Just like your high blood pressure or high blood sugar will return if you stop the medication, the weight can increase if you stop obesity medication. But this is the case with most drugs for chronic diseases.

The third objection is also correct. Why take drugs if diet and exercise will reduce weight? The fact is that diet and exercise does not succeed in each and every case. There are people who simply will not lose weight, no matter what. Obesity drugs are generally reserved for such cases. Your doctor can make the decision if you need such help. Mainly, these drugs help you feel less hungry or feel more full. This feeling by itself does not reduce weight. Instead, it empowers you to control temptations and enables adherence to weight-loss diets more effectively, thereby producing greater weight loss due to better compliance.

We have about 100 drugs for high blood pressure. This allows the doctor to try various drugs for their patients, till your doctor finds one or more drugs that suit you – drugs that your blood pressure will respond to. In comparison, we have only five obesity drugs that were recently approved by the FDA for long term use. This severely limits the choice of a physician in finding a drug that suits well for treating obesity for an individual. I hope that future will see many more obesity drugs that are even more effective and safe. This is very essential, if we are ever going to successfully address the global obesity epidemic.

Finally, a word about the role of diet / nutrition and exercise for those who are not overweight or obese. It is not enough to think of nutrition only to treat obesity. Good diet and exercise are equally needed for those who are not struggling with weight. For example, there seems to be a misunderstanding that you need exercise or walking only if you have the weight problems. Others are off the hook. This is not true. Exercise has many benefits for slim people too.

Likewise, you are what you eat. Good nutrition practices are essential for all. Even if you are not struggling with weight, it is a great idea to get some feedback on your diet pattern from a professional who can analyse your routine diet for you, give some feedback about what may be too much / too little in the diet and provide at least some general tips to improve the quality of your daily diet. This kind of proactive diet pattern analysis can help you with a timely course correction in your lifestyle, that may prevent a health issue in future. A stitch in time saves nine. This is one more of my dreams to see nutrition science being used pre-emptively to prevent disease and enhance health, in addition to using for disease treatment.

All in all, nutritional science fascinates me. I hope that you have received some health benefits of good nutrition through this book. Wish you happy reading and healthy living.

Acknowledgements

I have been fortunate to receive much love, affection and support from my family, friends and colleagues. I have immensely benefited by learning something from almost each and every one of them. Over the years, my teachers and mentors have contributed to my personal and professional growth in so many ways. I owe gratitude to Professors Sam Chang of North Dakota State University, USA, and Pushpa Kulkarni of Bombay University Department of Chemical Technology, for honing my research skills, and to Professor Richard Atkinson of the University of Wisconsin Medical School, USA, and my father, Dr Vinod Dhurandhar, for providing rare insight and understanding about the field of obesity. I am also indebted to my students, mentees, post-doctoral fellows and colleagues of our research team, who have helped advance obesity science with various cutting-edge discoveries over the years.

More specifically, I would like to gratefully acknowledge some individuals of who contributed to this book in some ways. At the outset, I should mention my wife Amrita, who is my soulmate, a sounding board for ideas and my ardent critique and best friend. Since I met her, I have no professional achievement that Amrita has not contributed to either directly or indirectly. From encouraging me to write this book, to developing the proposal, in editing my thoughts and writing, my son Rohan has worked shoulder to shoulder. There would be no book without his loving yet watchful involvement in the entire project. His wife and our daughter-in-law, Dr Emily Dhurandhar, who is also an obesity researcher and a leader in the field, has been a wonderful resource in developing many scientific aspects of the book. Emily is a third generation 'Dr Dhurandhar' in the field of obesity. I am hoping that their son, Armand, will take to obesity research, like his parents.

I would also like to express my heartfelt thanks to literary agent Kanishka Gupta for his very able and candid guidance throughout the process of book development, despite his busy schedule. His demand for perfection is infectious, and is easily reflected in the book. I would like to gratefully acknowledge the very engaged involvement of editors Debasri Rakshit and Shreya Punj, on behalf of HarperCollins *Publishers* India. The book has hugely benefited from their diligent and careful edits and suggestions. A huge thank you to Mr Aamir Khan, for being the inspiration for this book and for writing a superb and thoughtful foreword.

Finally, I wish to conclude by expressing my heartfelt thanks to my parents Dr Vinod and Late Anuradha Dhurandhar, and my brother Mihir, for their unconditional love in my life.

I have tried to cover and explain as many steps, tips and dietary advice needed for weight loss and weight maintenance in this book. To learn and do more, visit the website: www. dhurandhar.com

The website builds on this book to offer:

1. A free BMR calculator to easily find out your daily calorie requirements.
2. More diet plan options and recipes.
3. One-on-one interaction with me and my team.
4. My blog where you'll find more on losing fat, maintain weight and living a healthier life.